Conversations About Psychology
Volume 2

Conversations About

PSYCHOLOGY

Volume 2

Edited by Howard Burton

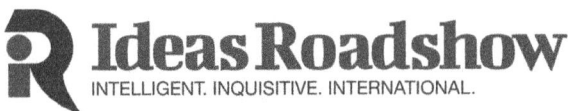

Ideas Roadshow
INTELLIGENT. INQUISITIVE. INTERNATIONAL.

Ideas Roadshow conversations present a wealth of candid insights from some of the world's leading experts, generated through a focused yet informal setting. They are explicitly designed to give non-specialists a uniquely accessible window into frontline research and scholarship that wouldn't otherwise be encountered through standard lectures and textbooks.

Over 100 Ideas Roadshow conversations have been held since our debut in 2012, covering a wide array of topics across the arts and sciences.

All Ideas Roadshow conversations are available both as part of a collection or as an individual eBook.

See www.ideasroadshow.com for a full listing of all titles.

ISBN: 978-1-77170-171-6 (pb)
ISBN: 978-1-77170-170-9 (eBook)

Edited, with preface and all introductions written by Howard Burton.

All *Ideas Roadshow Conversations* use Canadian spelling.

Contents

THE LIMITS OF CONSCIOUSNESS
A CONVERSATION WITH MARTIN MONTI

BEYOND MIRROR NEURONS
A CONVERSATION WITH GREG HICKOK

EXPLORING AUTISM
A CONVERSATION WITH UTA FRITH

Textual Note

The contents of this book are based upon separate filmed conversations with Howard Burton and each of the five featured experts.

Ellen Bialystok is Distinguished Research Professor of Psychology at York University and Associate Scientist at the Rotman Research Institute of the Baycrest Centre for Geriatric Care. This conversation occurred on August 21, 2014.

Victor Ferreira is Professor of Psychology at UC San Diego. This conversation occurred on April 12, 2014.

Martin Monti is Associate Professor of Psychology at UCLA. This conversation occurred on April 6, 2014.

Greg Hickok is Professor of Cognitive Science and Director of the Centre for Language Science at UC Irvine. This conversation occurred on September 26, 2014.

Uta Frith is Emeritus Professor of Cognitive Development at the Institute of Cognitive Neuroscience at University College London (UCL). This conversation occurred on September 2, 2012.

Howard Burton is the creator and host of Ideas Roadshow and was Founding Executive Director of Perimeter Institute for Theoretical Physics.

Preface

Psychology has changed considerably over its relatively brief but intensive history. From William James to Sigmund Freud to fMRI, a wide array of techniques, approaches and attitudes have come and gone as the prevailing wisdom has careened from dualism to behaviorism to behavioralism and beyond. But throughout all its manifold fashions and fluctuations, one dominant human characteristic has been consistently recognized as a fundamental key to penetrating the mysteries of our minds: language.

Language is both stunningly universal—no human society has ever been known to occur without it—and a clear mark of human distinction—no other member of the animal kingdom has ever been known to possess anything like the linguistic sophistication that humans exhibit. If there is such a thing as "the human condition", it is pretty hard to imagine it not having something strongly to do with language.

It's particularly fitting, then, that each of the five conversations included in this psychology collection have something significant to say about language.

Perhaps the most startling result is the groundbreaking work by York University psychologist **Ellen Bialystok** on the link between bilingualism and dementia. Ellen is an internationally-renowned researcher in the psychology of bilingualism and had previously discovered that the bilingual brain was far more likely to have stronger neural executive control networks that enable it to multitask better than the monolingual brain, but the correlation of bilingualism with dementia took even her by surprise:

"If you take a large enough sample—and it has to be a large sample, because these are widely, varying data—and you just look at the age at which people start to show the first symptoms of dementia; on average, the age at which the first signs of dementia are recognized is significantly older for bilinguals.

"The puzzle is that dementia, Alzheimer's disease, is initially a memory disorder. It's not a disease of executive control. How does an experience that boosts the front part of the brain protect against a disease that initially strikes the middle part of the brain? The memory disorders that are the first symptoms of Alzheimer's come from the hippocampus in the medial temporal lobe. How does being bilingual have any impact on that?

"The theory, yet to be confirmed, is that because the front part of the brain, this important area where we find this set of executive processes, is more efficient for bilinguals—more intact, has better connectivity, better grey matter density, and so forth—it's better suited to provide compensation. The front part of the brain is kind of domain-general: it's not used for just one thing. In other words, having a robust front part of the brain can somehow carry you through as deterioration is happening elsewhere. It comes in as a kind of reserve."

But you don't have to study bilingualism to get big surprises. UC San Diego psycholinguist **Victor Ferreira** demonstrates that even our naive picture of seemingly straightforward linguistic communication within one language has some unexpectedly big problems with it.

"We feel as though our job as speakers is to construct sentences that are as easy as possible for the listener to understand. So if I have a choice between one that's easier or more difficult for my listener to comprehend, the system presumably was designed, or has evolved, to choose the easier one, thereby making me better at my job of having the listener understand me. But, in fact, that's not the case.

*"But as it turns out, ambiguity and difficulty for the speaker are probably largely independent of one another. It's not that I actually **aim** for things that are potentially ambiguous because that will be easier for me, it's that I'm not paying attention to certain forms of*

ambiguity when I'm trying to put a certain, what we call prosody, on my sentence: where I lengthen certain phrases or shorten certain phrases because that could serve a disambiguating function.

"The reason that our original intuition, according to this framework, is perhaps incorrect, is because it turns out that, as a speaker, I've got a pretty big job to do all on my own. As a speaker, every time I formulate a sentence I have to come up with the message that I want to get across. We call that message formulation. I have to search my vocabulary—which has between 30,000 and 80,000 words, depending on exactly what you count as a word—for just those words that will work. I have to figure out the correct grammatical ordering of those words so that I convey who's doing what to whom, and it's a valid grammatical structure in my language. I have to figure out how to sound out the words. And I have to figure out how to impose the right prosody on the sentence. All this at a rate of about two to three words per second, so 300 milliseconds per word.

"When you formulate the computational problem that way, I think it goes some way towards illustrating the difficulty of trying to perform additional tasks."

UCLA psychologist **Martin Monti**, meanwhile, illustrates how an intriguing hypothesis on the nature of language processing can be falsified, tangibly demonstrating how the accumulation of scientific knowledge continues so long as some clear result is obtained.

Intrigued by the apparent structural similarity between certain linguistical and mathematical expressions, Martin naturally wondered if this might be a sign of something deeper going on in our brains.

"A very simple example that I've used in a slightly more elaborate form is to look at the sentences "John kissed Mary" and "Mary kissed John". These two sentences have a similar relationship to '5-3' and '3-5'.

"Exactly the same tokens in each of these expressions have a certain position, and the specific position occupied allows us to infer

meaning. Within each pair, the meanings are extremely different: who's the agent—who's kissing whom—and which number is getting subtracted from the other and so forth. And the question to me is, The fact that we recognize this difference, the fact that we're sensitive to the position in which tokens appear in these expressions, is this a consequence of our ability for language? Does this ability in math, for example, this ability to understand the difference in meaning between 5-3 and 3-5, somehow derive from our ability for language?

"*We've actually tried to measure this empirically, by testing healthy volunteers. We put them in an fMRI machine and we took pictures of the metabolism of their brain while they were using their language faculties to understand the relationship between different tokens in a sentence; and we took pictures of their brain while they were solving similar problems, but now in math.*

"*Now, the question is—at least the way we frame it—if our sense of syntax in math comes from the sense of syntax in language, we ought to see the same parts of the brain that you use to understand syntax in language be engaged when you're thinking of these related algebraic problems.*

"*It turns out that that's not the case. The parts of your brain that you use for language naturally apply to language, but they do not get used for the similar task in the domain of algebra.*"

Our last two examples highlight how our painstakingly-acquired understanding of the science of language might be harnessed to shed light on many other areas of frontline cognitive science inquiry.

UC Irvine speech and language psychologist **Greg Hickok** describes how his extensive, specialized knowledge of the field served as an immediate trigger to provoke suspicions that the wildly fashionable "mirror neuron" hypothesis that was taking the international cognitive science community by storm could not possibly live up to its billing:

"*I first heard about mirror neurons in a lecture that Giacomo Rizzolatti gave—I think it was at the Cognitive Neuroscience Society meeting in San Francisco. It was fascinating. There were these cells that were responding both when the monkey was generating actions and observing actions, and everyone was interested. It was starting to gain some steam. That was back in the early 2000s, I believe.*

"But I ignored it. It wasn't relevant to my work at all. I had no interest in it. Even though the mirror neuron folks were claiming that it had relevance to speech, I knew it couldn't be the case, because of a condition known as Broca's aphasia.

"It's been known since the 1860s that when you damage the frontal motor speech circuits, you can disrupt the ability to produce speech quite severely, while not necessarily impairing the ability to perceive or understand speech or language.

"So I thought at that time that, while maybe the mirror neuron story held for monkeys and their actions; in terms of speech—my area of research—it just didn't pan out."

Lastly, University College London autism expert **Uta Frith**, speculates how rigorously exploring the overlap between language and so-called "mentalizing" could one day enable us to more meaningfully distinguish between two rather different types of conditions that both lie on the so-called "autism spectrum".

"I know exactly what the classic autistic child should be like as originally described by the psychologist Leo Kanner: the child who has this aloofness, isn't connecting to this world, and who also has some stereotyped behaviours—he's very rigid and also some kind of relatively outstanding ability.

"Now that package I recognize. The question is: 'Is that package due to the same kind of underlying processes that produce this? Or is it a sort of coincidence?' I say a "sort of coincidence" because I've actually rejected the idea that it's a complete coincidence. But at any rate, we just don't know yet: we don't know yet whether this is a particular subgroup about which we should say, 'OK, that's the Kanner type.'

"The Asperger type is actually very similar except it seems all much milder, much more to do with good language while the Kanner type has to do with bad language—on the whole, very, very impaired language. Again, people say: 'Why don't you explain that specifically, this impaired language?' And you could say: 'OK, that's another add-on: it's a superimposed thing that you happen to get.'

"You're on this hazardous developmental path: one thing has gone wrong already, another thing has gone wrong. Now we come to language: that could be going wrong in many different ways too. We've tried to explain the language difficulties in terms of lack of mentalizing but that doesn't fit with the Asperger-type where language problems don't occur but the mentalizing problems do."

It's a fool's game to speculate on what the next big breakthrough in psychology is going to be. But one thing is certain: if it doesn't significantly increase our detailed understanding of how we use language, then it's probably not that big after all.

The Psychology of Bilingualism

A conversation with Ellen Bialystok

Introduction

The Plastic Revolution

A long-running debate in the linguistics community is centered around something called the Sapir-Whorf hypothesis, after Edward Sapir and his erstwhile student Benjamin Lee Whorf, two famous linguists who first formulated it most explicitly in the first half of the 20th century. Loosely put, the question is whether we experience the world around us through whichever language we happen to speak (as Sapir and Whorf believed), or if our mental "world views" are fundamentally language-independent.

In other words, does language shape our thoughts? Or do our thoughts—the product of some underlying cognitive processes common to all—shape our language?

As the battle raged on, Ellen Bialystok, Distinguished Research Professor of Psychology at York University and Associate Scientist at the Rotman Research Institute, has neatly sidestepped the issue by looking at something slightly different. Ellen is one of the world's most foremost authorities on the measurable effects of bilingualism on our brains: *what objective differences, on average, can be detected between those who speak two languages, as opposed to just one?*

Somewhat surprisingly, perhaps, it turns out that there are a good deal more differences than we might, at first, have suspected.

The first major distinction that Ellen appreciated concerned something called "metalinguistic awareness".

"The most important linguistic achievement for young kids is developing what is called metalinguistic awareness: knowledge about

language, understanding what language is and that it can be manipulated. If you don't understand that language is a structured system, you can't learn to read, because you can't figure out that the things on the page refer to something in language. So metalinguistic awareness is crucial.

"In the first studies that started in the late 1970s and continued for about a decade, a number of people, including my own group, were looking at the development of metalinguistic awareness and finding that, by and large, bilingual children are ahead. The bilingual kids were developing these metalinguistic insights up to a year earlier."

Bilingual children, then, through their experience of regularly manipulating two languages from a very early age, develop a faster appreciation of the structure of language itself.

Well, that's interesting, but perhaps not very surprising. And anyway, does it really matter? After all, just because bilinguals get there faster doesn't necessarily mean all that much if we all get there eventually.

But then Ellen started noticing other things. It seems that, on average, bilinguals—both children and adults—performed decidedly better on standardized tests involving a large amount "cognitive interference", when the subject was deliberately subjected to misleading information. These tests can be verbal (like the famous Stroop test, where subjects are asked to identify words like "green" based on the colour of their ink, which is typically changed to a range of different colours) or non-verbal (such as measuring reaction times of dots on different sides of a screen with different hands).

This was progress, then, of a sort: it seemed the bilingual brain really *is*, objectively, at least a bit different than the monolingual brain. The problem, though, was to determine if this scientifically demonstrated difference was any more societally relevant than simply being able to do better on a few arcane and largely irrelevant psychological tests.

So Ellen and her colleagues starting imagining how these differences might be more generally manifested in the real world. After all, if bilinguals were somehow able to, on average, insulate themselves against misleading or extraneous information, then surely we should be able to see evidence of this in other places than simply the Stroop test.

And yes, indeed, that turns out to be the case. Through a number of cleverly-designed experiments, it was discovered that bilinguals, on average, performed objectively better at a series of diverse tasks— from driving while on a cell phone, to cooking many items simultaneously—all of which involved an ability to successfully multitask, simultaneously filtering in and out different streams of information.

But that was only the beginning. Ellen, who began her scientific career as a developmental psychologist studying language acquisition in young children, then began looking to see if the effects of lifelong bilingualism might somehow manifest themselves in the elderly, specifically examining those who suffered from dementia.

In a series of groundbreaking studies, Ellen and her group demonstrated that the first signs of dementia are typically delayed a whopping 4–5 years for bilinguals compared to monolinguals. Bilingualism is no cure for dementia, it needs to be stressed, but somehow the bilingual brain is able to significantly delay the impact of severely debilitating diseases like Alzheimer's. Follow-up research using fMRI brain-scanning technology revealed that bilingual brains tend to have a slightly different neurophysiology—more grey matter and white matter—than their monolingual counterparts.

Talk about hugely relevant research. We are, suddenly, a very long way indeed from measuring differences in reading words in different coloured ink.

And yet, puzzles abound. What, for example, is happening in the brains of bilingual people that enable them to more successfully battle against the ravages of Alzheimer's disease?

Ellen believes the answer lies in a specific region of our brain called the prefrontal lobes. Modern brain scans have shown evidence that bilinguals have a better prefrontal lobe network that, in turn, directly enables higher levels of executive control. And it is this boost in executive control that allows them to mask the effects of dementia better than monolinguals.

> *"The theory, yet to be confirmed, is that because the front part of the brain, this important area where we find this set of executive processes, is more efficient for bilinguals, it's better suited to provide compensation. The front part of the brain is kind of domain-general; it's not used for just one thing. In other words, having a robust front part of the brain can somehow carry you through as deterioration is happening elsewhere. It comes in as a kind of reserve."*

That sounds plausible enough. But how did these enhanced networks get developed in the first place? How can the very act of speaking two languages change the very structure of our brains?

> *"What we now understand about the brain is that it is massively plastic. The brain is not a fixed framework of rigid connections, but is a dynamic, plastic system. It molds itself on the basis of what you're asking it to do, and the more you train your brain, or require your brain to do certain kinds of things, the more it will reroute your neural circuitry to reflect those experiences, which means that the brain is a strong reflection of your experiences.*

> *"If you think about it that way, it's not so surprising that something as pervasive as the language, or languages, that you speak is going to rewire your brain. People are surprised that bilingualism rewires the brain. They think it's crazy. But it isn't crazy at all. Everything rewires the brain."*

And suddenly, from a rather unforeseen direction, a bright light shines on our old conundrum of whether language shapes our thoughts or thoughts shape our language.

The solution, neuroplasticity tells us, is quite simply yes to both.

The Conversation

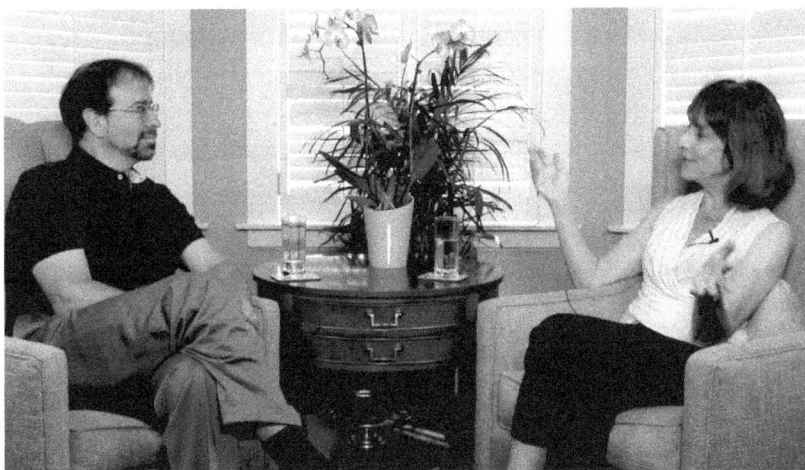

I. Focusing on Bilingualism

From pedagogy to battling stereotypes

HB: How did you get involved in bilingualism research? How did that start for you?

EB: It was a natural extension of the research I was doing. In research, you don't really know where it's going to lead. One things leads to another and then you follow up the questions that are left over.

I was studying language and cognitive development in children. That's what I did for my graduate work. I was interested in how children learn language and how that connects up with their developing cognitive systems, and things evolved naturally from there.

When I graduated, I ended up working on a project that looked at second language learning in high school classrooms, something there was very little research on at the time. This was the 1970s. Kids were learning languages in high school and nobody was really paying much attention to it.

HB: What were you looking at, exactly—how quickly kids were able to pick up another language?

EB: This was in Ontario, so we were looking at kids learning French in school. Is there any point to it? Does it do anything for them? Do they actually learn French? Does anything actually happen?

It was part of a large-scale project that examined matters very much from a pedagogical perspective. It was housed in the Faculty of Education, and the questions all had a natural educational orientation: *How should we teach language? What are effective strategies for teaching? What are effective strategies for learning?*

It was all very much at the level of pedagogy—which was something I knew nothing about, by the way. But I knew something about language, and I knew about aspects of language development in children, so I was hired to manage a part of that project.

HB: And what did you find out?

EB: We found out almost nothing, as it happens. Many of these big, pedagogical questions had no real answers of the sort they were looking for—a kind of one-size-fits-all answer.

HB: But were there not even micro-results? Something along the lines of, *If you do this particular thing on a regular basis with this built-in control group, this tends to work statistically better than that?* There was nothing at all?

EB: Nothing of any interest, except that some kids were learning French and some kids weren't—but that, in itself, is interesting.

There was also, at the time, a wider interest (including the group I was working with) in discovering what they were calling the "good language learner". Some people claim to know 26 languages, all fluently, and some people cannot learn to say 'bonjour'. They cannot do it. Their whole being rejects that. So what's going on here?

There were a few studies that tried to figure out what it is that enables some people to be good language learners, as opposed to others. Again, those studies didn't show much, but I now actually have an opinion on this.

I have a very holistic view of the mind, brain, and ability. In my view it's dead simple: everybody's good at some stuff and bad at some stuff. Just like every other activity, learning a language is a kind of talent. Some people are very good at physics, or math, or music, or dance, or sports, and some people are very good at language. We all have some sort of an ability profile, and if you link up ability with interest, motivation, and opportunity, you'll learn language. I think it's pretty much that simple.

HB: Of course, we all learn language. There's a question about how much of it is innate and how much of it is learned, but there's clearly a large, innate component to being able to learn language.

EB: Well, in some sense, everything we learn is innate because we are innately prepared to learn it. But I would put this question out there: *do we all learn our first, and perhaps only, language in the same way, to the same level, with the same degree of proficiency?* I don't think so. We're not all poets. Everything is distributed. Some people just love language and they learn it easily—they eat it for breakfast. If you give them more languages, they'll eat more breakfast. And some people end up being pretty rudimentary in their linguistic abilities. Even there, there's a distribution, I think. Of course, we're wired to learn language. That doesn't mean the *content* of language is innate. It means the *ability to learn* this content is innate.

HB: Getting back to your story, you were doing these pedagogical studies, and recognized that they were somewhat less than ideally efficacious. What happened after that?

EB: Well, what that did was introduce me to this world of, at that time, pretty nascent research in second language acquisition. Within that very small area of research, there was an even more nascent crumb that looked at second language acquisition from the perspective of psychology. I thought, *Well, now I'm on to something, because I was trained as a psychologist,* so I just gravitated to that. There were a few people—a very small number of people whom I could name on one hand—who used the methods of psychology to look at these questions in more detail. And I became one of those people.

We started asking questions about this from the perspective of psychology. *What's the mind doing when you're learning another language? What's happening to the language you already know? How do they live together? Does something else change? How can we, as adults, take on a whole new way of speaking?*

These are psychological questions, not pedagogical questions. There were a small number of us who started asking those questions.

Finally, not only was I trained as a psychologist, I was trained as a developmental psychologist. So I ended up asking those questions from the perspective of children's development.

HB: By children, you mean mostly younger children?

EB: Yes—at first, mostly younger children. That set out the first stage of my research: what happens to children's language and cognitive abilities when they are learning or have been exposed to two languages in the home?

HB: You had written in one of the review papers that, up until the early 1960s, there was a prevailing societal view that children who were bilingual, or at least had competency in two languages, had all sorts of negative, developmental aspects associated with them as a result, and it wasn't until this famous study—

EB: Peal and Lambert in 1962.

HB: Right—that some serious research started to be done to correct our understanding.

But first: where did this notion come from: that people were somehow developmentally handicapped by having two languages?

EB: I think it came from two places. The first is that people are afraid of language, and the second is racism. The combination of these things was lethal.

I should add that, even though the conclusion was pretty terrible—"languages are bad", "protect your children from other languages"; these are the kinds of things people would say—there was a little bit of research that fed right into that conclusion. This research had been done with the best of all intentions, except that it was badly done and it came out with the wrong results.

At any rate, people are afraid of languages, especially in North America (much less so in Europe, though Europeans are not immune to these attitudes). But certainly in North America; and particularly in the 1950s when all of this was becoming popular belief, people thought, *Language is very hard. I'm so glad my child is learning to speak English on schedule. I'm not going to mess with that and confuse them with another language, because we know that, when we look at kids who have to speak two languages, they just mix them all up and they don't know which language they're speaking. It's too hard and I'm going to protect my child.*

Everybody wants the best for her child. So this was an honestly motivated, well-intentioned opinion that just happens to be wrong.

HB: Sure. But it's not a scientific opinion.

EB: No, it's not. And it's based on anecdotal evidence. In fact, it's true that if you take three-year-old kids who are raised in homes where two languages are spoken, they will mix up the languages, but not because they're confused. It's actually quite brilliant, what they're doing. What they really want to do is communicate, so they will use all the resources they have, and if they don't have a word they need in one language, they're just going to use what they know from the other language, because they're motivated by communication. An adult might mistakenly respond, *"Oh, this is shocking. He used the French word and he's supposed to be speaking English."* But it's actually not shocking—it's quite reasonable.

Questions for Discussion:

1. Can a love of language be stimulated? If so, are we, as a society, doing a sufficiently good job of stimulating it in our children?

2. What are some of the current sociological stereotypes we have about language acquisition?

II. Becoming Scientific

Inklings of plasticity

HB: This leads us right into the studies. Let's talk about what you and others found.

My sense is that, until that 1962 paper by Peal and Lambert, by and large there weren't many rigorous, empirical studies that were conducted. From that point onwards, there started to be a basis of scholarship and studies that you've certainly contributed to. Can you tell me a little bit about those studies and what sorts of things you and others found?

EB: The way we started was by looking at language abilities. Bilingualism is a linguistic experience. If you're going to find any effect, you'd think it's going to be in something to do with language.

The most important linguistic achievement for young kids is developing what is called *metalinguistic awareness*: knowledge about language, understanding what language is and that it can be manipulated. If you don't understand that language is a structured system, you can't learn to read, because you can't figure out that the things on the page refer to something in language. So metalinguistic awareness is crucial.

In the first studies that started in the late 1970s and continued for about a decade, a number of people, including my own group, were looking at the development of metalinguistic awareness and finding that, by and large, bilingual children are ahead. The bilingual kids were developing these metalinguistic insights up to a year earlier.

HB: How do you measure that?

EB: We use different tasks. I'll give you an example of one that we've used to great satisfaction. It's a simple, silly task, but it has given us great insights. Any linguist will tell you that what a native speaker can do is intuitively tell you if a sentence is grammatical or not. If I say, *"The orchids are on the table,"* you would say, *"Yes, that's how you'd say it in English."*

You can do this even with very young children who are just learning English. Children as young as three years old can tell you if a sentence is grammatical or not; and we put a little wrench in it by asking them to tell us if the sentence is said the right way, even though the sentence might be a little silly. We give them all the permutations, and then we come to sentences like, *"The orchid is on the nose."* And they may say, *"The orchid is on the nose? That's ridiculous. It's on the table,"* to which we'd reply, *"Yes, but is that sentence said the right way?"* What you have to do is separate the grammatical structure from the meaning. That's the essence of metalinguistic understanding.

HB: They have some appreciation of the structure of grammar without focusing on the semantic content.

EB: They understand that the two are separate. And bilingual kids tend to gain that awareness earlier.

We even have evidence now, using brain imaging, that even bilingual adults make the distinction better than monolingual adults. They'll all get the right answer, of course, but you can see what's going on in the brain of a bilingual adult, and it shows that they can do it better than the monolingual adult.

HB: So the first studies you were doing, the studies we were just talking about, were these metalinguistic studies.

EB: Exactly. So we got that clear. It's not terribly surprising that using two languages means that you understand the structure of language better.

The next step, then, is to say, *"Well, what else is going on? Is the rest of the mind involved in this?"*

Here, I have to say, there's an assumption that people still hold about the brain. I read an article in the *New York Times* a while ago about the biggest myths about the brain that people have. One of these assumptions people have is that the brain is divided up into little sections, and that we only use some of them, and that there's all this specialization. Well, that's not true. We use all of our brain. The brain is just one big blob that has specialized wiring within it, so everything affects everything.

HB: Moreover, there are plasticity issues that come into play, which hopefully we can talk about later.

EB: Yes, we'll definitely talk about that, because that's key.

Just in terms of how it functions, what you're doing with language has to affect what you're doing with everything else. We were actually the first group that struck out and said, *"Let's look at the rest of cognition,"* although this was anticipated by the Peal and Lambert study: the idea that you can find differences in just ordinary cognitive measures that aren't necessarily linguistic.

We were then able to look at kids who were monolingual or bilingual and give them tests of cognitive ability to see if there was any difference. The important thing we found is that, if you just give kids tests that look like intelligence tests, or knowledge tests, or anything like that, the performances of bilingual and monolingual kids is exactly the same.

But if the task involves some kind of conflict where there's misleading information, like the sentence, *"The orchid is on the nose"*, where you have to just ignore the meaning so you can look at how the sentence is said. If you translate that to some non-verbal task, where you have to ignore something that's pulling your attention, the bilingual kids were better. What they were able to do is focus on what's important without being distracted when two things are competing for their attention, and we found this to be the case for non-verbal tasks as well. That was the next step in studying how bilingualism was affecting the mind in more general terms.

Questions for Discussion:

1. Have you heard the expression that "we only use 10% of our brains? Where do you think this idea comes from? Do you think that there's any merit to it at all?

2. Can the amount of metalinguistic awareness be somehow quantified rigorously? If so, how might that work?

III. Out of the Minds of Babes

Focusing attention from the earliest moments

HB: My understanding of what's going on is that when a bilingual child is engaging in the world, both in a verbal and a non-verbal way, these two systems, these two languages, are both, at some level, working simultaneously. Even if the child is operating in English and is English-French bilingual, the French cognitive functions are still happening, so there's this sense that the child is able to turn one off or dim one down and focus, because they have this added experience of navigating through a situation with different information flows. Is that a fair way to look at it?

EB: That's exactly right; and I'm going to make it a little more complicated by telling you about some very recent evidence, which people have reported, showing that you can find these effects, these advantages in paying attention to one thing and shutting out distraction, in the first year of life. People have looked closely at kids who are raised in homes where they're hearing two languages and discovered two key results. These are babies, seven months old, who can't speak a single word, but are hearing two sources of linguistic input. It was found that, first of all, they know exactly which language is which; and second, when you then take those babies and give them a very simple, baby attention task, where they have to focus on a toy or something like that, they outperform monolinguals.

All of this happens very early in development, then, and you don't even need to be able to use the language. For all of this to be put in place, you just need to have two sources of input that are setting up two systems that the child understands are separate.

HB: Let me try to be very concrete to see if I understand what's going on. My understanding is that the strategy that the children would be using to identify representations of objects would be different if they had this bilingual sensitivity. So if I'm a kid who is raised in a bilingual home, the idea is that I know, at some level, that the word 'glass' pertains to that specific object, but there might be other words that also pertain to that same object; whereas, if I'm somebody who is monolingual, I just assume that that one word pertains to only one object. Is that right?

EB: That's what we used to think, but that's intellectualizing it too much, because that isn't going to explain what's happening in the six- and seven-month olds.

That's what we used to think the case was for older kids. For example, a three-year old knows that he can call the object 'the glass', or '*le verre*', or whatever. That's what we used to think, but these findings with infants take it down a notch, because infants are not really figuring out word-to-object mappings: they're just figuring out these two systems.

And if you want to *really* raise the stakes, take neonates just a few minutes after birth who were in utero in a monolingual or bilingual environment. They too showed different familiarity responses to the languages they heard *in utero.* How's *that* for pushing the boundaries?

HB: That's remarkable. But how do you actually do those studies? How do you set up the experiments?

EB: Infant research is a very special thing, and I don't do it—it's way too hard. But in any kind of research that you're doing, you have to exploit the responses that your subjects are able to give you. If you're doing research with rats, for example, you're not going to set up a verbal task; you're going to set up something that rats can do, which might be learning to run a maze for a food reward, or something like that.

Similarly, with infants you have to set up something that infants can do. And what infants can do is show familiarity or not. If you present a new stimulus, a new sound, or a new sight, they'll show you through their expressions whether something is interesting to them or not. They habituate very quickly. This is how we know how infants decide what things are the same.

For example, if you want to know if an infant can see the difference between a circle and a square, you hook the infant up to a computer that has a sort of pacifier attached to it, and when the infants are excited, they suck furiously, and when they get bored they stop sucking, or the sucking diminishes. So you keep doing this until the infant is totally bored with what she's seeing. Then you change the stimulus from, say, a red square to a red circle. If the infant can tell the difference between the square and the circle, she'll think, *This is a whole new thing! Now it's a circle!* and the sucking increases, so you know they've seen the difference. If it doesn't increase, you conclude that they don't recognize the difference. You exploit what infants do.

That's the kind of method you would use to figure out if these very young infants see two languages as being, first, the same or different; and second, familiar or not.

HB: So in practice, then, you would speak to them in different languages and see if their stimulation rate would increase as you switch the languages or if they wouldn't be able to tell the difference.

EB: Yes. I don't do those experiments, but that's the basic paradigm.

The study that I'm thinking of was done with infants who were born either to mothers who were in completely English, monolingual, environments, or to Filipino mothers who, during pregnancy, were in environments where both English and Tagalog (a primary language of the Philippines) were spoken. After these babies are born, the researcher presents them with either English, or Tagalog, or a third language—which, I think, in these studies, was Japanese—that none of the infants had ever heard.

Questions for Discussion:

1. How might Ellen's remarks to Howard about "intellectualizing too much" be related to the difference in the way adults and children learn language?

2. What, if anything, do the infant studies mentioned in this chapter tell us about the innate nature of human curiosity?

IV. Differences and Definitions

Statistically significant results, and defining bilingualism

HB: As a non-specialist, I'd like to point out some things I read that struck me as interesting. As I understand it, if you look at children who are bilingual and you measure their vocabulary using various testing methodologies and compare their ability to that of a child of the same age who is in a monolingual environment, the bilingual child would, indeed, statistically have a smaller vocabulary in any one of those languages than the monolingual child would. Is that correct?

EB: Yes, but I want to add a very important qualification. It is statistically correct to say that the vocabulary of a bilingual, in one of their languages, on average, is smaller than that of a monolingual speaker, for the one language that they speak. We've shown that statistically with very large samples. We have two studies published with almost 2,000 children and almost 2,000 adults, which both show that. So that's *statistically* true. But what does it really mean? You have to be careful about the interpretation.

We get vocabulary scores from standardized tests. Any standardized test that's properly constructed will give a normal distribution across the population with a mean, in these cases, of about 100, because that's how they've been standardized.

The first important point is that, when we give these vocabulary tests to our very large samples, we get exactly a normal distribution. That's a very important point. What happens is that that center mean point for the monolinguals and bilinguals shifts slightly. On average, the monolinguals we test are about five points higher than the population average, and the bilinguals we test are about five points lower than the population average, and that's highly significant.

But, as you can imagine, with these two normal distributions that just shift slightly, there's a huge amount of overlap. Most of the time the curves overlap, and that means that, for the majority of people in those distributions, it can go either way. Many bilinguals are going to outperform monolinguals on the vocabulary test. You have to be clear about a statement that's true for populations, and a statement that's true for individuals.

HB: Sure. I'm not implying that, if you're bilingual, you're necessarily not going to perform as well as a monolingual.

EB: But people do interpret it that way.

HB: Okay, so it's important to clarify that, as you say. But, still, from a scientific perspective, it's a significant result.

EB: Yes, it is.

HB: There are all sorts of reasons why that might be the case. My understanding is that you've speculated that if, let's suppose your parents speak English at home and you go to a French school, you would be exposed to all sorts of words that are in a scholastic environment, but you might not be aware of words for things that you find around the house. There are all sorts of possible reasons.

But it is a statistically significant result that argues (at least statistically speaking) that it is somewhat disadvantageous to be bilingual in terms of one measure—the statistical likelihood of just knowing more words in one particular language. However, that is compensated for by various advantages, such as the metalinguistic aspect you mentioned earlier.

There seems to be this idea of interference and focus. Can you talk a little bit more about that, as well as some relevant experiments?

EB: If we pick up the story where we left off with those early studies on kids, our next question was whether bilingualism had any enduring value. The tasks that we were giving kids to do in those early studies, where we showed that bilinguals were solving these tasks better—these were all things kids were going to do eventually anyway. By eight or nine years old, all the kids could do them. Maybe the bilinguals just got there a little sooner. So what?

The next stage in the research was to look at adulthood and aging. We started by just taking tasks from the cognitive literature where performance assesses the ability to resolve conflict: the simple idea of interference. You see two stimuli, say, and you have to figure out how to pay attention and ignore distraction.

A very good example, and a task that's often considered to be the gold standard of this sort of interference control, is the Stroop test, created by John Ridley Stroop in 1935.

The idea is that the researcher shows the subject words and the subject has to say the colour of the ink. Perhaps they may show the subject the word 'blue' written in blue ink, and the subject says, *"Blue,"* or the word 'red' written in red ink where she naturally responds, *"Red."*

However, if you take the word 'blue' and you write it in red ink, then the idea is that you have to say that it's red, not blue. You have to just focus on the colour of the ink, not read the word. Now you've got two different things that are pulling you.

It's like the example I mentioned before: *"The orchids are on the table"* sounds alright; *"The orchids are on the nose"* doesn't. Well, you want to say *"No,"* but you have to focus on the structure and say, *"Yes"* instead. The Stroop test is exactly like that. You want to read the word and say *"Red"* or whatever the word happens to be, but the rule is that you have to name the colour of the ink.

This is a prime example of what bilinguals are doing.

If I am a French speaker, say, who wants to say, in English, *"The glass is empty"*, I must focus on *not* saying *"Le verre est vide"* in French instead of English. It's the same sort of thing. On tasks like that, the Stroop task being an example, we found that adults and older adults who are bilingual, show less effects of interference.

HB: Again, it's this idea that they're so used to these two systems happening at the same time, and they're so used to shutting one down, or toning one down, that, in other tasks that are similar, where they have to do that, they've already had the experience, or had their brain adapted, or whatever—hopefully we'll get into the brain a little later.

EB: That's right. It's something that they find easier to do. It's simply less effortful.

HB: Again, this is an empirical study, a scientific result that allows you to say, *"People who are bilingual are, on average, better at doing this."*

EB: Yes.

HB: Before we continue, I'd like to make a small diversion. We're throwing this word 'bilingualism' around, and I'm wondering, *What does that actually mean, rigorously?* Can you define it? We all have some intuitive sense of what it means, but I would imagine that there's a fairly wide spectrum of what we actually mean by 'bilingualism'.

EB: That's a really important question. The question about who is actually bilingual is key to all of this research, and the answer is not simple. Some people have taken a very pragmatic approach and say, *"Let's just say that anybody who has the ability to communicate in two languages is bilingual."* This is the approach taken by a psychologist in Switzerland named François Grosjean.

As you say, almost everybody has some experience with other languages. What's really rare is complete monolingualism. How many people haven't experienced any other language at all? The question is, at what point does your familiarity with another language move you into a different place?

We like to think about it as a spectrum, and there are two principal ways we've used this notion of a spectrum in our research. The first is, if we really want to say that bilingualism as an experience has very specific outcomes on the mind and brain, then the best way to go about getting evidence for that is taking the clearest cases. So we deliberately select people whom we consider to be the most bilingual.

We then have very high standards that they have to meet: they have to have been exposed to two languages from early childhood, they have to use both all the time to a high level, and so forth. Those are really clear endpoints. So we compare those people to people who, say, had to endure high school French but then never spoke it; we would generally consider them monolingual. If we take very clear cases, then we can compare the two groups and say what bilingualism is.

However, as you said, bilingualism is, to some degree, all the stuff in the middle as well. So in other studies, we don't classify people by groups; instead, we quantify people for where they are on the scale, and then we use a different kind of statistical approach to see if position on the scale is related to position on an outcome.

Question for Discussion:

1. Do you agree with the statement that "anyone who has the ability to communicate in two languages is bilingual?"

V. Multitasking and Focusing

Real-world applications of bilingualism's advantages

HB: So there's the Stroop test, and the Simon test, and so forth, that are used to evaluate these things. I understand why psychologists are doing this: they're looking to conduct measurements in a controlled environment to determine if there's an objective difference between different categories of people. So they make empirical measurements based on how quickly certain types of people can identify whether something is a circle or a rectangle, or in blue or red ink, and all the rest of that. But at some level, I'm thinking, I don't really care about that, because I'm not doing those tests in my regular day-to-day life. What difference does all that make to me?

What I'm most concerned about is whether or not being bilingual gives me some advantage or predisposition towards doing something in the real world. Can I say, for example, that the reason Roger Federer has so many Grand Slam titles is somehow related to the fact that he speaks all sorts of different languages—or that his bilingualism is, at least, somehow beneficial to his ability to concentrate? Can we say anything about that sort of thing at all, even at a speculative level?

EB: You're exactly right; and I'm going to go further and say that, to a large extent, these tests that we use in the laboratory are really a bad approach. The reason they're a bad approach is because they're too specific: the effects are too subtle, and they assume that what you're doing when you're performing a Simon task, for example, is really connected to the more important questions that you're talking about. So I agree completely.

As laboratory scientists, these are largely the tools that we have. But I'll give you two examples where I think we were able to go a little further, because you're right: when's the last time you were walking down the street and somebody stopped you and said, *"Howard, you have to stop right now and do a Stroop test before I let you cross the street"?* It doesn't come up a lot. However, other aspects of life really require those abilities. I'm going to give you two examples.

About 10 years ago, I was involved in a PhD study from a lab that worked on driving safety. It was a very practical, applied psychology set of questions about how people negotiate safe driving, and they had a driving simulator in the lab—not my lab, as it happens, but a colleague of mine who does this research. One of his PhD students had the idea for his dissertation that we have all this data now about how driving with a cell phone is really a bad idea, so he wondered, *Is it worse if you're driving while talking on a cell phone and you're speaking in a second language?* And that's how I got involved.

We ended up doing a study and, as tends to happen, I kind of corralled it more towards my interests. The heart of the study ended up being this: he had a driving simulator, and he brought in people who were monolingual or bilingual—these were all young adults—and he gave them all these tasks in English. The bilinguals were people who spoke another language at home, meaning that English was probably their second language. But they were all university students, so their English was fine.

Then he said, *"We're going to do two things. First, I want you to sit at this table and perform a bunch of verbal tasks."* They were the sorts of things you need to do when you're having a conversation, like repeating back sentences, defining words, and other simple, verbal things. Then he said, *"Now, put that all aside and sit in the driving simulator, where you drive this course and get a score for how many times you crash and how safe your driving is."* Then, he put it all together. Now the subject is told to sit in the driving simulator and do the verbal tasks all over again. Basically, he had them driving while trying to produce coherent language.

The first thing to say is that everybody is terrible. Make no mistake: it's really a bad idea to drive while talking on your cell phone. Everybody's safe driving scores were significantly worse when they were doing the verbal tasks, but the bilinguals were not as bad as the monolinguals.

This is the thing: it's about multi-tasking, and that experiment was an example of multi-tasking in the real world. You have to divide your attention so you have enough of it on the road when it needs to be there and enough left over to carry on a coherent conversation. The point is that even though there's an overall decline in your safe driving score, it's a significantly less severe drop.

The second example comes from a task that we created called "the breakfast task". It's this complex, virtual-reality thing, where you have to make breakfast by cooking five different foods that all take a different amount of time to cook, and you have to have them ready at the same time—something that I find utterly impossible to do in real life, as it happens. You have to know when to start and stop these foods; and just to make it more complicated, while you're not monitoring the food cooking, there's this table-setting task where you have to set as many place settings as you can, and you get a score for how many place settings you manage to squeeze in while cooking these foods. Moreover, the recipes for these foods are all on different pages—it's very complicated. So you get scores for everything: how accurate the stop times are and other things.

But one of the crucial scores is a switching score. If you're setting the table and trying to get that last knife and fork in place, and suddenly the eggs need to be turned off, are you able to disengage and go over to the eggs? That's the essence of switching: you see that your attention has to be shifted.

We did this with older and younger, monolingual and bilingual adults. On all the cooking scores, they were exactly the same. But the bilinguals were better at switching. They were setting more tables and they were not stuck at the table when they should have been turning off the eggs. They were multitasking in a way that the monolinguals weren't—even though, overall, their basic performance scores were the same.

That's what these processes in the brain do. These attention-shifting and inhibiting functions of the brain actually have a real-world implementation. And on the couple of examples that we've been able to demonstrate, the bilinguals really were better.

HB: I'm guessing you're going to find, as you think about this even more and develop more tests, that this is even more pervasive than we had imagined. There's a huge amount of things that we do in our everyday life that is part of the spectrum of multitasking.

I'm wondering too about looking in the other direction. We're talking about multitasking, and making sure that you can do things simultaneously, and switching, because, again, as I understand it, the theory is that people who are bilingual have these parallel processes going on all the time. But what if we looked at it the other way in terms of one's ability to concentrate or focus on one particular area? Might it be possible that people who are monolingual are better at being able to focus for prolonged periods of time? Have any tests been done in that particular way?

EB: I don't know of any studies that show that, but I'm not convinced that monolinguals would be any better. At any rate, we're almost never in a situation where there are no distractions. Think about what happens in the real world. Think about a kid in a classroom; a classroom is an utter noise machine. How a kid can focus attention on a blabbing teacher or a boring textbook when the whole environment is conspiring to distract them—that's the real challenge in the real world. In the real world, what bilinguals are doing has a very important application.

HB: And the need to successfully multitask is presumably increasing considerably these days.

EB: I think we naturally adopt strategies that make our world simpler. As somebody who would qualify as an older adult according to the criteria in my own experiments, I know that I consciously multitask less because I can't do it anymore. I know that I used to be able to have three things on my mind at the same time, but I can't anymore, so I consciously reduce.

We have an interesting result. In that breakfast task that I described, we also ran another condition where we brought in older adults who had Parkinson's disease. One of the consequences of this disease is, in fact, a deficit in these exact processes: there's an executive function deficit and multitasking is harder, which naturally made us wonder what would happen.

We had a group of Parkinson's patients who were age-matched and cognitively-matched with our monolingual control group that I described. We gave them the breakfast task and, to our utter amazement, these people were getting cooking scores as good as the young adults. They were doing as well as the young adults on stopping and starting all these foods. How is this possible?

Well, it turns out that, probably completely unconsciously, they had a strategy. They simplified the task. They ignored the table. They only went to the table when they were absolutely sure that there was nothing else they needed to be doing. They took a complex, multitasking environment, reduced it to something they could manage, and they did it very well.

HB: Because they had to do that. They had trained themselves to be able to do that, just to survive, given the constraints that Parkinson's had imposed on them.

EB: Right. They adapted. I'm sure it was not conscious, but that's how they adapted to their limitation.

Questions for Discussion:

1. Has your ability to multitask increased or decreased over the past five years? Why might this be the case?

2. Do you agree or disagree with the claim that there might be a link between an increased societal need to multitask and a general reduction in concentration ability?

VI. In The Brain

What's happening inside

HB: Let's talk now about what's actually going on in the brain. I've held you back from talking about that, but I really want to discuss the networks involved and what might be happening neurophysiologically.

So we have this theory, as I understand it, that people who are bilingual or multilingual have different processes going on in the brain which enables them to multitask better, which enables them to filter things out and make better judgments in real time given all of these constraints.

The question is, what does that mean neurophysiologically? What's actually happening in the brain? And what do we think is happening in terms of the networks for, not only language, but cognition in general, for both monolinguals and multilinguals?

EB: I think the first thing to say is that what we now understand about the brain is that it is massively plastic. The brain is not a fixed framework of rigid connections, but is a dynamic, plastic system. The brain molds itself on the basis of what you're asking it to do, and the more you train your brain, or require your brain to do certain kinds of things, the more it will reroute your neural circuitry to reflect those experiences, which means that the brain is a strong reflection of your experiences.

If you think about it that way, it's not so surprising that something as pervasive as the language, or languages, that you speak is going to rewire your brain. People are surprised that bilingualism rewires the brain. They think it's crazy. But it isn't crazy at all. Everything rewires the brain.

Now we can ask, *in what way* does it rewire the brain? I think the answer rests on the observation that you've now made a few times: because there are always two systems available for every linguistic and cognitive interaction that we engage in, the brain has to figure out how to direct attention to the right one.

It does this, I think, by invoking the basic, general system we have that's part of the basic structure of the brain. We have, in our brain, a specific system that is involved in conflict resolution. Every time there's conflict and you have to decide where to go, we invoke what we call *the executive control system,* or *the executive function system,* or *the prefrontal lobe network.* That's the system I'm referring to here—it's there to guide our attention.

Bilingualism is always challenging our ability to attend to the right thing and not get misled by the wrong thing. That frontal system gets involved, gets wired in, from the very beginning, to linguistic networks, to cognitive networks and to semantic networks. The whole brain of the bilingual person is wired with more distribution across the hemispheres as well as front to back, so it's a more distributed brain network; and, crucially, it makes far more use of the frontal systems than would otherwise be found in monolingual brains.

HB: My understanding is that this is all very plausible based upon what we know about the frontal lobe, executive control, and all the rest of that. There has been a wealth of empirical research done on this using brain-scanning devices, fMRI, and so forth. Presumably, you've actually seen real evidence of this.

EB: Yes, and the newest evidence, which is coming out now, is even more impressive because it's structural: that is, it looks at brain structure.

There are a couple of labs now—two notably: one in London and one in Milan—that are showing that, if you actually measure cortical thickness (the amount of grey-matter neurons) in those frontal regions, bilinguals have more. Bilinguals have greater cortical density in crucial, frontal regions.

We have published evidence showing better white matter for bilinguals. White matter is the myelin that covers the neurons involved in the communication network between different brain regions. Brain cells communicate by signalling to each other, and they get covered with this white tissue that speeds up the connection. It's kind of like a fibre optic system. So, the thicker and more intact that myelin is, the better this communication system works. And we have evidence showing that, in older bilinguals, the myelin on the fibres that go from the front-right side of the brain to the back, and then across the corpus callosum, are more intact

Questions for Discussion:

1. Why do you think it took cognitive scientists so long to appreciate the brain's inherent plasticity?

2. What might the specific mechanisms for neuroplasticity be? How might tests be developed to distinguish between different possible mechanisms?

VII. The Art of Measurement

The power of fMRI

HB: Describe what's going on in these experiments. How do you do them, exactly?

EB: The way the technology is set up right now is really brilliant, because you can get all sorts of information all at once. In an ideal experiment now, you have a participant in a fMRI scanner where the fMRI has the capability of making a structural image of the relevant tissues. There's a functional coil that will reveal the brain activation that's occurring while the individual is actually performing a task, and there's another coil that measures the integrity of the white matter structure. So you get functional information about what's connected to what—you get information about the grey matter structure (the actual architecture of these brain regions), white matter structure, and now, very interestingly, you get information about what the brain is doing functionally at rest. This is really new, leading-edge stuff.

People have now identified these networks. So when you're sitting there with a clear mind, not thinking about anything, there's still connectivity. And, it turns out that that connectivity is extremely powerful in predicting cognitive ability and performance.

So the brain at rest tells you a lot about how the brain is organized and what it is capable of doing. There are a couple of these at-rest networks that are particularly related to executive control performance; and there are some that aren't.

We now have evidence comparing older monolingual and bilingual adults (these are 72-year-olds), and we have images of their brains showing these networks at rest. These people are told to lie in the scanner and look at a blank screen; and the only instruction is to not fall asleep.

What we see is that, for certain kinds of these rest networks— like those responsible for memory or vision—the groups are exactly the same. But in terms of the two networks that are known to relate to performance in executive control, the bilinguals have better connectivity at rest, which means that their brains are simply more prepared for these processes.

HB: And have you done studies, or are you planning on doing studies, that evaluate these networks in people who have learned languages at different stages of their lives? Have you compared people who were exposed to different languages *in utero*, say, to those who began learning a second language much later in life? I'm guessing there might be different levels of activation of these networks across that spectrum.

EB: The research is still too new to know if that's what would happen. But my intuition is that that's exactly what we'd see, because these are all spectrums that arise through training experiences. The effects come through practice, so I would expect that, if you were able to conduct these studies in sufficient numbers with sufficient control, you would find a relationship between how much bilingual experience the individual has had and how these networks are aligned. That would be my expectation, but we're a long way from having enough data to know if that's the case.

HB: I'm also wondering if it might be possible to go the other way. Here's what I mean by that. Granted that if I speak two languages, I will have a characteristic network in my brain that is used for various different functions, and that I'll have a greater emphasis on the executive function in my frontal lobe than somebody who is monolingual. So might it be possible to take someone, train them using means other than language learning to develop the same sort of executive function, and then, as a result of that training, somehow give them an enhanced ability to learn a second language? The idea would be that you would somehow be predisposing the brain to learn a new language. I understand that there's no causal link between having those networks and learning a language (it's the language training that causes those networks to be enhanced in the first place), but it seems at least logically possible that it might somehow make it easier to do so.

EB: Some people actually argue that. There is actually an argument that it goes the other way around.

HB: OK, but I'm not saying that.

EB: But some people argue that, so I'll just put that argument out there. Some people say, *"No, executive control allowed this person to become bilingual. It's completely the other way around. What you have is variability in executive control. Those people who had high executive control were therefore able to learn another language and they became bilingual."* Some people do make that argument.

HB: Well, alright. But that's clearly silly.

EB: Thank you for saying that.

HB: It's clearly silly because you obviously have many people who become bilingual simply as a result of circumstances.

EB: That's what I argue. But, while we're still on this digression, I should mention that those who argue that then go on to say, *"Well, we have evidence that executive control is necessary for second-language learning, especially in adulthood."* And it is, of course (executive control is necessary for lots of tasks), but I would like to just dismiss all of this because it muddies the waters.

To take one concrete example, we had some trouble with what I think was a fabulous paper that was held up in review, because one of the reviewers insisted that you need executive control to learn a language in the first place. And this is ridiculous, because the paper was exactly what you're going for: it's a training study.

We took monolinguals and we gave half of them a year of Spanish classes and then we looked at their brains. We thought, *What could be cleaner?* But this reviewer was holding things up by insisting on this one point.

HB: OK. For my part, I'm interested in this notion of plasticity and what you can do with it, and whether the arrows only work in one direction, or whether they go both ways. Everything we're doing is affecting the neural architecture in terms of how these systems evolve and what they do and how they exist. I think that can be very liberating for a lot of people, because they have this sense that nothing is written in stone and they can consistently develop.

EB: I would be happy to agree with that if the point were clear enough. Usually I think about it a bit differently: I think about bilingualism as being accompanied by release of all of this energy that then enables the person to do other things. But recent circumstances have made me be a little more cautious. It can get a bit messy.

Questions for Discussion:

1. To what extent does it make sense to talk about the brain "at rest"?

2. Is there a difference between "the brain" and "the mind"?

3. Would your interest in learning another language increase if you believed that doing so would have other "side benefits"?

VIII. Bilingualism, Extended

The challenge of isolating relevant factors

HB: Here's a different question entirely, then. I'm listening to you tell me all these wonderful things that happen if my child is bilingual. Maybe I want to make sure my child is super-fantastic, so I decide to teach them 10 languages, or even 20 languages. Is that reasonable? Is there an upper bound to the benefit of learning additional languages? Are there diminishing returns with regard to the effect on these networks and strengthening this executive control function?

EB: The question about whether more languages are better, is interesting—and, I think, possibly intractable. First, I can say that there are several studies out there. Some show that multilingualism is even better than bilingualism, while others show there's no difference.

But I think there's an inherent problem in even asking the question, and the problem is this: When we compare monolinguals and bilinguals, I can be pretty sure that, except for how many languages these people end up speaking, most other things in their lives are pretty much the same. They are just as smart, they've had similar educational opportunities, and in every other respect as far as those things go I can say that they're pretty much the same. Then I can conclude that, if the outcomes of some specific test are different, then it must be a result of bilingualism.

But I think when you move into multilingualism, you are pushing the edges of that assumption. As I said earlier, just like other activities, people are different in their language ability. People who have a particular talent for language may be the ones who go on and learn many more languages. Perhaps learning languages requires a lot of time management, a lot of education. Or maybe there are other factors at work. Maybe people who go on to multilingualism are just smarter or had better opportunities. When you study multilinguals, you lose the ability to assume that nothing else is different. Once you've given up on that, you don't know what's causing the result.

Questions for Discussion:

1. Does learning one language make it easier to learn another one?

2. To what extent does learning additional languages impact one's ability to speak one's native language?

IX. Bilingualism and Dementia

Surprising results and current puzzles

HB: Let's talk about dementia. You've done some really seminal work on this and had some really quite astounding results. What, specifically, have you found out about the link between bilingualism and dementia?

EB: The result is very simple. If you take a large enough sample—and it has to be a large sample, because these are widely, varying data—and you just look at the age at which people start to show the first symptoms of dementia; on average, the age at which the first signs of dementia are recognized is significantly older for bilinguals. We've shown that several times in our sample, which has—very gratifyingly—been replicated in many different places around the world.

HB: And this age difference that you're talking about is something like four to five years, right?

EB: Yes, it's a significantly large difference. But it has to be that large because, if it were less, it wouldn't be significant because the variability is so huge.

When we did the first study, the one that was published in 2007, the results were really striking. In that study the age difference we found was four-and-a-half years. I remember thinking, *How is this possible?*

In that study we had about 100 monolinguals and 100 bilinguals, and the bilinguals were about four-and-a half-years older, on average, when they first started demonstrating signs of dementia. But what's astounding is that the range of first evidence of dementia begins in both language groups at 45-years-old and then goes right up to very late in life. These are huge ranges. Unless there is a pretty large difference between the mean onset age in both language groups, you're not going to get a statistically significant result, because there's so much variability.

That was the first study, but we've replicated it about three times. It's been replicated in California, in India, in Belgium, in lots of places now. This is clearly a real effect. Someone who has been a lifelong bilingual can mask the effects of the early symptoms of dementia for a significant period of time.

Now, four or five years, as you pointed out, is a huge difference; but it's even more important in this situation than it would be if we were talking about a disease that could strike only between the ages of, say, 30 and 35. Because dementia is primarily a disease of aging, if you can buy four or five years, it's a game-changer. This has huge implications for public health, family, quality of life, and so on.

HB: So what's going on, exactly, neurophysiologically? Is it that this masking can occur because the dementia affects this executive control function in the frontal lobes, and, therefore, the individual has more experience in being able to use those networks to somehow compensate? Or is it something else, you think?

EB: The puzzle is that dementia, Alzheimer's disease, is initially a *memory* disorder. It's not a disease of executive control. How does an experience that boosts the front part of the brain protect against a disease that initially strikes the middle part of the brain? The memory disorders that are the first symptoms of Alzheimer's come from the hippocampus in the medial temporal lobe. How does being bilingual have any impact on that?

The theory, yet to be confirmed, is that because the front part of the brain, this important area where we find this set of executive processes, is more efficient for bilinguals—more intact, has better connectivity, better grey matter density, and so forth—it's better suited to provide compensation. The front part of the brain is kind of domain-general: it's not used for just one thing. In other words, having a robust front part of the brain can somehow carry you through as deterioration is happening elsewhere. It comes in as a kind of reserve.

HB: That's not so surprising, given the importance of that part of the brain combined with what we know about plasticity, the fact that the brain can be modified in so many different ways.

And in terms of concrete effects, my understanding is that there are two ways that this manifests itself empirically. The first is some statistical aspect which involves comparing the age at which dementia has been diagnosed for these individuals and then cross-matching that with their linguistic capabilities, as you've just said.

But there's another way of measuring this as well, I understand, which is to look at people at the same stage of diagnosis and compare their brains using various scans; and it turns out that those who are multilingual actually have greater pathological aspects to their brains—which implies that, exactly as you're saying, they're able to mask the effects of their dementia better than the monolinguals.

EB: That's right. We have one study that showed that. We have another study where we do not have brain data, but we have data on their performance levels, and it feeds into the same story. We would like to be able to do more detailed brain studies to confirm those ideas, but, right now, that's the main data we have.

Questions for Discussion:

1. *What does Ellen mean, exactly, when she says, "Yes, it's a significantly large difference. But it has to be that large because, if it were less, it wouldn't be significant because the variability is so huge?"*

2. *How might we more rigorously define, and experimentally probe, Ellen's notion of "cognitive reserve"?*

X. Public Policy Implications

The societal benefits of bilingualism

HB: I understand that you're not in the public health field, nor are you the President of the United States or the Prime Minister of Canada, but if you *were* in a situation to direct public policy, what sorts of recommendations might you have, given your knowledge, regarding the benefits of multilingualism?

EB: Well, I think the benefits of multilingualism for a society go well beyond what I'm talking about here. We've been discussing individual advantages: the benefits that might accrue to me personally if I'm a bilingual individual. But on a societal level, the effects are far greater still.

The greater the openness that societies have to multilingualism, the better the society for all sorts of reasons: socially, politically, and so forth.

Societies that are open to bilingualism are better off for a whole host of reasons. They are more open, tolerant societies. They're more culturally diverse. They're more engaging. They respect lineage by enabling children to communicate with their grandparents who may speak a different language. Everybody wins if language is accepted as a wide value in society.

Some people ask, *"Well, if bilingualism has these effects on dementia, then, at a societal level, is it the case that bilingual societies or cultures should have less Alzheimer's disease than monolingual cultures or societies?"*

That's absolutely not true; and it's not true for many reasons.

First, because bilingualism doesn't prevent Alzheimer's disease. We know that. But also because you can't compare across societies.

Societies have different health systems, different education levels, different social conditions, different socio-economic configurations. Everything is different.

You can't take the result from an individual and plunk it into a society and say, *"If only Canada had better French education so that everybody would be bilingual, we would have some sort of a bulwark against dementia."* That's not the societal implication of my work, or anyone else's.

What we're talking about here has to do with social values: what we think is important for society, why we think it's important for kids to learn other languages. In Toronto, for instance, and in many parts of the rest of Canada, we consider it very important for people to be able to keep their heritage language as the language of the home and have that language respected by the community, so that shops down the street and local media will provide services in that language. This is as opposed to other countries where that will not happen, where only the official language is respected or accepted.

None of these issues are about the cognitive implications of bilingualism, they're about the social implications. But people might be more accepting of those ideas if you can connect them to the fact that it's also good for people's brains.

HB: So in the opposite way to when, pre-1962, people had this notion that bilingualism was bad for your brain, now you can say that it's a good thing for all these other reasons—and, by the way, it also happens to be very beneficial to the brain.

EB: Exactly. And that's actually the direction of argument that I prefer. I think that the social arguments are the really powerful ones: they're the reasons people should be paying attention and policy-makers should care. And, by the way, it's good for your brain.

Questions for Discussion

1. Do you think that, on average, multilingual societies are more open and tolerant than monolingual societies? How might such a claim be tested?

2. What do you think are the dominant factors that lead people to be fearful of their society becoming multilingual?

XI. Open Questions and Speculations

Ongoing mysteries and the problem with projections

HB: Getting back to the research side of things, let me now make you an offer. If I were an omniscient being and I could answer any scientific questions you might have, what would you ask me? I'd like to know what's keeping you up at night, what you're most puzzled by, what you're most excited by, what you're most curious about.

EB: Well, there are a lot of questions.

This is hard research to do because it's messy. What I try to do in my research is—to use the phrase from Nate Silver—take the signal out of the noise. You get all kinds of variables and it's all very messy, and you have to try very hard to understand what the signal is telling you. I would like greater closure on this.

We think we know how the brain is being modified by this intense experience, but if we could understand better what's happening as people learn and use languages, and thus figure out how brains evolve in real time, in a real ecology, we would have tremendous access to how the brain works. That is, use language as one of the roots to understanding how the brain works. Because in spite of what some people will tell you, the brain is still largely a black box. And as much as some people claim that we have it figured out, mostly we don't.

Because language is our most prevalent experience, it's the most human of our experiences, it could be one of those lenses through which, if we get it right, we may be able to figure out more about how the brain works. That's one kind of question I wish we had better insight into.

The other question I would ask is more on the behavioural side, and relates to a point you've raised a few times. Bilingualism is messy. If we could figure out more about what the mess is around the bilingualism and the people we study, and the mess around the tasks we use, we could understand these effects better.

Many people, including us, run experiments. We use people whom we think are monolingual or bilingual, we use tasks that we think are getting at the right thing, and we don't get any useful results. It doesn't work. Lots of experiments just don't work. What's the difference between those that don't work and the ones that do? Knowing that would help us understand more clearly what the interactive conditions are.

Both from the brain side and the behaviour side, we need to somehow reduce the mess. I think if we could do that on this one problem—how do bilingual brains work?—we could get a better understanding—in general, overall—about the mind and brain, simply because language might be the most important thing that the brain does.

HB: I'm going to ask you to speculate now. Granted that we're at a very preliminary stage in terms of developing a comprehensive understanding of the brain (notwithstanding the hype that some people may be putting out there), at what point in the future do you think we'll start getting a genuinely deeper understanding of these concepts? We've made remarkable progress in all sorts of ways, in terms of the technology and the associated research that has been accomplished.

The field of psychology has changed remarkably over the past 30 years, not only because of this advanced technology, of course, but it has certainly been strongly influenced by the technology. It's very difficult for me now, as an observer, to draw a line between psychology, neuroscience or cognitive science. All these things are kind of mixed together. More specifically, you naturally tilt to the linguistic side of things as well.

If I were to ask you, "When will we have—however you'd like to define it—a genuinely deep understanding of these core issues?" what would you say? 50 years? 25 years?

EB: I would not put a number on it, but I'll give you some perspective on how it's going. As you say, the changes are remarkable and they are exponential, not linear; that's very key. Once you're on an exponential scale, projections become wilder because you don't know.

I'm thinking about what I used to hear with regard to projections of when the entire human genome would be mapped. When it was finally mapped, the astounding thing was that it took significantly less time than all the projections, because once they got the basic stuff figured out, the advances they made were exponential, and what they ended up with was simpler than what they expected. There were just fewer genes than they were expecting to find. So that was a game changer too.

When you're projecting about the unknown, you just don't even know what the factors are. So I wouldn't make any guess in terms of numbers, but I would say that progress is being made at an impressive rate and the insights make sense. That tells me that things are moving in the right direction.

HB: And, specifically, what future work are you involved in right now, or are you thinking about doing over the next couple of years?

EB: What I'd love to do more of in the immediate future is to look at the brain underpinnings of the dementia results that we've had. I would love to be able to figure out what's different between the brains of monolingual and bilingual patients with dementia, because then you can project backwards and understand how they got there in a much clearer way.

HB: This gets back to what you said before about how it's possible that the executive control functions in the frontal lobe can affect the hippocampus and other areas.

EB: Exactly.

HB: Well, thank you very much. This was a pleasure.

EB: Thank you.

Questions for Discussion:

1. Are you surprised by Ellen's comment that "Lots of experiments just don't work"? Does this give you more, or less, confidence in the scientific process?

2. Will increasingly accurate brain-scanning technology eventually render traditional "behavioural psychology" obsolete?

Speaking and Thinking

A conversation with Victor Ferreira

Introduction

The Tip of the Tongue

UC San Diego psychologist Victor Ferreira makes a habit of paying attention to revealing little things that most of us routinely overlook.

For example, examine the following two sentences: *The teacher knew I was going to be late* and *The teacher knew that I was going to be late*. What's the difference between them?

Not much, it seems, other than the innocuous "that" in the second sentence, which grammarians call a complementizer. But for Victor, Principal Investigator at UCSD's Language Production Lab, this seemingly inconsequential "that" is little short of a linguistic gold mine.

The decision of a speaker to introduce, or not introduce, a "that" often has little effect on the difference in meaning between two phrases, so deciding whether to include or omit it seems to carry little to no consequence in terms of meaning.

> *"What's valuable about the fact that there are sentences like this is that the word itself is practically meaningless. It's very inconspicuous, but nonetheless the fact that the sentence requires that you have mentioned it (or not) means that your brain made the decision:* **Yes, this sentence requires a "that"** *or* **No, this sentence won't have a "that".**

> *"I almost see it like a linguistic drosophila—it's our fruit fly. If I can figure out what the factors are that compel a speaker to say a "that" in a sentence—or not—that's going to tell me something about how our sentence construction mechanism works."*

So what has this linguistic drosophila done for us, exactly? Well, in a series of experiments, Victor and his colleagues have unexpectedly demonstrated that, in normal discourse, speakers aren't nearly as focused on expressing things clearly as we might have naively thought.

It turns out that, in many instances at least, the speaker opts for constructions that are simply easier to say rather than easier to understand.

This may seem pretty selfish until we begin to appreciate all the complexities involved in the everyday act of normal speech production.

> "It turns out that as a speaker, I've got a pretty big job all on my own. Every time I formulate, say, a 7-word sentence, I have to come up with the message that I want to get across; search my vocabulary—which typically has between 30,000 and 80,000 words—for the correct 7 words; figure out the correct grammatical ordering; figure out how to sound out the words; figure out how to impose this prosody on the sentence... And all of this at a rate of between 2-3 words per second. So there's a lot going on."

Far too much going on in most cases, it seems, for speakers to also be concerned with rigorously weighing up a spectrum of possible expressions to choose the one that best conveys their intended meaning.

So that's a most interesting result. But even more impressive is the process, how linguistic researchers have devised ingenious ways to probe just how the brain's speech and language functions operate.

And according to Victor, this is just the beginning, as modern brain-imaging technology has done little less than revolutionize the entire discipline.

> "It's really clear at this point that the fields of behavioural science, broadly speaking, and cognitive science specifically, are going through a kind of a neural revolution. The degree to which neuro-science techniques are going to be important for doing investigations

of cognitive functions is increasing, and it's just going to become more and more important."

So we have vastly improved tools to test our theories these days. But what sorts of theories do we actually have?

"There are a number of factors pointing us toward a belief that our language knowledge is, in fact, shaped by ongoing experiences in a way that we hadn't quite appreciated before.

"There's a whole new line in cognitive science that has risen to prominence the last 10 or 15 years that views a lot of what human beings do as optimal. The common thread in a lot of this research is to take some instance when a human was seemingly behaving irrationally and show that, in fact, he's behaving rationally when you take into account all the other factors that might be relevant.

"In the language sciences this has been unfolding in a way that suggests that the way we understand language, the way that we produce language, isn't just some fixed grammar that gets into our head and stays that way. Rather, by responding to contingencies in our environment, our language system will change and adapt.

"It's almost a tuning argument. So my lab is moving in this direction as well. We're spending more time looking at what are the ways that you can show that there is some learning event that happened in your recent past that's now going to change the way that you end up describing something in the future."

According to this view, then, it's not just that individual languages evolve in response to environmental stimuli, but so does our very capacity to produce and use language in the first place.

It's a very big idea that, at first glance, seems miles away from the business of rigorously examining when someone might slip in a "that" or not in a sentence. But the beauty of experimental science is that many seemingly innocuous features of the system often turn out to be highly significant—indeed, many core aspects of our modern theory of language production came about through carefully studying speech errors in the 1970s.

For linguistics, then, just like many other disciplines, the devil is very much in the details, and carefully combing the subtleties of speech may well prove key to revealing the pivotal cognitive mechanisms of how the brain processes language—and, along the way, shed some deeply revealing light on what makes us human.

The Conversation

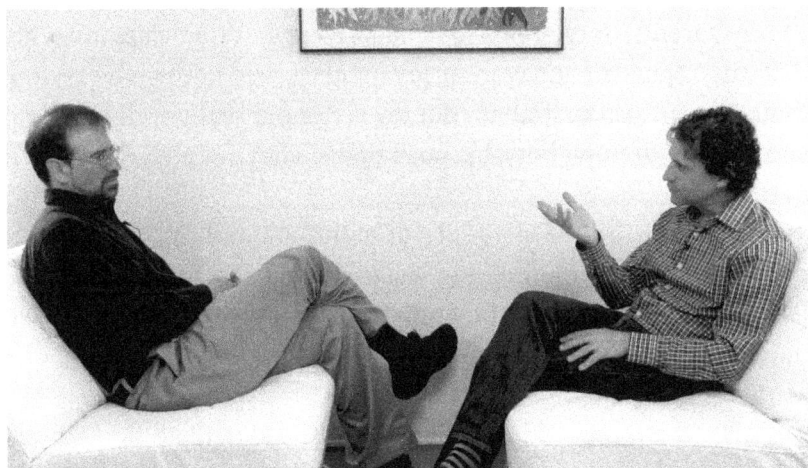

I. Linguistic Beginnings

In search of relevance

HB: You told me earlier that your sister was an inspiring figure for you in psycholinguistics. How did she inspire you, exactly?

VF: My parents, immigrants to Canada, were working-class folks. My dad was a construction worker. My mom worked both in the sewing industry and as a custodian. But my sister did really well in school so she went to university, because that's what people who do well in school do.

She went to the University of Manitoba and did an honours project with a psycholinguist there named Murray Singer, who is a prominent figure in the field of text comprehension: how we understand passages of text and how we draw inferences from one sentence to another.

After the project, he suggested that she should go to graduate school because she was a natural at it. He advised her to apply to the University of Massachusetts at Amherst, which was one of the strongest schools in the world, especially in reading and eye-tracking. So she went to UMass Amherst and also worked with another leading researcher named Chuck Clifton.

She finished up her PhD in 1987 and then took a job at the University of Alberta. This is just as I was finishing up high school.

HB: Was this a postdoctoral fellowship or an assistant professorship?

VF: She went straight to an assistant professorship.

HB: Okay. So she's an Assistant Professor in psycholinguistics at the University of Alberta and had this very accomplished beginning to her career, but how did that affect you and your career? Presumably you looked up to your sister and were inspired. Was that it? Or was there also something else involved?

VF: Well, it's how these things often go. Let me give you a quick aside. I used to teach the honours seminar in our department, and for part of the junior seminar we would ask the faculty members in our department—and other departments, if they were doing related work—to come in and tell us about their research so that the honours students could hear about it and potentially work with them on their honours project.

As an ice breaker I would ask all of the people coming in to tell us their story of how they got into their research. It's very useful for the students to hear how people get interested in what they're doing. And what's remarkable is that at least seven out of ten stories involved serendipity.

There was one guy named Mike Cole, who was in the Communications department here at UCSD (he's retired now) and is one of the leading people in the Vygotskian approach to language and communication. He does what he does because he got out of an elevator on the wrong floor. The elevator doors opened and there was a flyer in front of him that said—this was 1960 or something like that—"*Go to Moscow!*" And he thought, *Go to Moscow in 1960 during the USSR? I'm not missing that chance!*

HB: I don't know anything about Vygotskian methods. Does it have anything to do with elevators?

VF: No, nothing to do with elevators. But he went to Moscow, learned this approach, and became one of the United States' leading researchers in this area. So many cases are random like this; and my case is kind of like that too.

In high school I pictured that I was going to be some sort of a scientist one day and took AP physics and chemistry courses. But right when I was taking my AP physics exam, I had a life crisis. I was solving some physics problem—calculating the electrical field in a solenoid or something like that, doing the right-hand rule— and I remember thinking to myself halfway through solving this problem on the AP exam, *I don't care what the electrical field is inside this solenoid. I really don't.*

HB: Right in the *middle* of your AP physics exam?

VF: Right in the middle of the exam. So I finished the exam and I did all right. But that's when I decided that I didn't want to do something like physics or chemistry because they seemed quite impersonal.

HB: It was nothing about solenoids in particular? You're not an anti-solenite or anything like that, are you?

VF: Not as far as I know. They're as interesting as anything else, which is to say, interesting from a precision standpoint. It was a situation where you could measure things and characterize them very accurately. That's part of what's very admirable about hard sciences like physics. But I just didn't feel it was quite as relevant or interesting to me as other subjects.

Around the same time, my brother-in-law also became a cognitive scientist. His name is John Henderson. He does vision science.

HB: Is there some sort of rule in your family that you have to go into this field?

VF: It's always explainable. My sister and brother-in-law met in graduate school at UMass. He was finishing up his thesis when he and my sister came to Canada, to Winnipeg, for a Christmas holiday. He was reading through his thesis document, and I was this little kid trying to check out this guy who was potentially going to be marrying my sister.

So I asked him, "*Hey, what are you working on?*" And he replied, "*Well, I'm working on my thesis.*" Then he explained his thesis, which was about using an eye-tracker to do skilled reading, and I thought,

*This is amazing. You can actually do scientific research on **people**?* I thought that science was about—

HB: Solenoids.

VF: Yes, exactly: solenoids. High schools don't typically have experimental psychology courses or cognitive science courses. They might now, but they certainly didn't when I was going there.

So that was my first exposure to the science of behaviour. I thought it was kind of interesting. Then I had my crisis incident during the AP Physics exam.

In the meantime, I had applied to college. At many Canadian universities—and McGill was certainly one of them—you apply directly to a faculty. I had applied to the faculty of science, so I knew I was going to do something in the scientific area.

The next thing that happened was that all of us—my sister, my brother-in-law, me, my mom—were on a vacation together. I had this course catalogue with me—they used to print them out in those days—and was thinking about the courses to take in the coming year.

My sister, who was then a beginning Assistant Professor at the University of Alberta, did what I would do—and what you would probably do—when she saw the course catalogue: She said, "*Oh, let me see that*," ripped it out of my hand, flipped to the psychology section, and said, "*You've got to take this course and this course*". She recognized some names and would say, "*This is a great person. You should try to take a course from him or her.*"

At that time my sister went to a conference—one that I now go to every year, in fact—and she bumped into one of our colleagues who was then a professor at McGill (he's now at the University of Wisconsin in Madison). She said, "*Hey, my little brother is at McGill and he thinks he might be getting interested in psychology. Is there any chance he could volunteer in your lab?*" My sense is that, as a favour, he said, "*OK, sure. Why not? You're a colleague.*"

She sent me an email. I remember getting it on one of those old terminals. It said, "*Mark Seidenberg is interested in having you as a volunteer in the lab. Why don't you go talk to him?*" So one day

I timidly knocked on his door. I was expecting him to say, *"Here's a bunch of data for you to code. Go through this and do a bunch of grunt work."* That would have been perfectly reasonable. But what he said was actually, *"Here are three papers that I want to do a project on. Go to the library, get these papers, and read them. When you're done reading them, come back."* I suspect he thought I was never going to come back again, but I did.

I went to the library and photocopied the articles. I remember calling my sister while I was reading these articles and asking, *"What are all these statistics? What's this F thing?"*

Then I knocked on Mark Seidenberg's door again and he said, *"I'm thinking about doing a study that goes like this,"* and he basically had me set up the study. It was quite remarkable.

HB: Did he do this with everyone, or was it just because of your sister?

VF: I don't know the answer to that question. Back then I don't think it was common for an undergraduate student to knock on your door and say, *"I want to be in your lab."*

HB: The studies were about what exactly? What sorts of things?

VF: Mark studied—and still studies—what we call word recognition. It's almost like pattern recognition when it comes to reading individual words.

For example, I might show you the word "pint" and ask you to read it aloud. I would time how long it takes you to do that. I know very precise properties about that word and I might try to link the properties of the word to how long it takes you to say the word aloud. "Pint", for example, is a word that is relatively hard to say because it's not pronounced how it should be pronounced. We know the way it's really pronounced, but given its spelling, it should be pronounced so that it rhymes with "hint" and "mint". The existence of "hint" and "mint", both of which are pronounced in that different way, actually slows your ability to pronounce "pint" the right way.

That was kind of along the lines of the study that he wanted me to do. He wanted to do a study based on the work of Robert Glushko. Mark wanted me to follow up on some studies that Robert had done on analogy and word recognition, the idea that maybe part of what you're doing when you're recognizing a word is based on analogies to other words.

HB: And all this while you were still a freshman?

VF: Yes, from November of my freshman year onward. And it was all mainly because, as I said, my sister bumped into this guy at a conference and said, *"Do you mind if my little brother volunteers in your lab?"*

So I started by doing that project with him. I actually don't think the experiment worked.

HB: But that gives knowledge as well.

VF: That's true. That's knowledge as well.

As a kid, I played around with computers a lot. In 1982 or 1983 when personal computers started to appear, I learned how to program: first BASIC, then Pascal, then C.

I started helping out the grad students in this lab, and a specific issue came up. They were doing word-recognition experiments where a subject would see a word and read it as quickly as they could, over and over again. I was helping somebody set up an experiment and I said, *"These words all appear in the same order all the time. That doesn't seem like a good idea."*

HB: Sure, because you're priming people.

VF: Right. And you might get carryover effects: if the first word is hard, that's going to make you slower on the next word even though it has nothing to do with the next word.

I said, *"Shouldn't the words be in random order?"* And the grad student responded, *"Yes, they should be; but the program we're using can't do that."* A little while later, I said, *"I know how we can do this.*

We can write a front-end program that generates randomly ordered lists and then feeds that to this program."

I suspect that what happened at that point was that the grad students got together with Mark Seidenberg and said, *"This guy has got some skills that might be kind of useful in the lab. I think you should keep him around."* So I ended up working with Mark the whole time I was an undergraduate.

In fact, it got a little more interesting than that. He left for the University of Southern California halfway through my time as an undergraduate. Back then, NSERC, the Canadian funding agency, offered undergraduate research scholarships for $2,000. Mark said, *"Get one of these NSERC undergraduate fellowships and I'll fly you down to Los Angeles for a summer and we can do work down here."*

HB: That's some serious motivation.

VF: Yes. So I applied, and happily I got it. He flew me down to LA and I got to hang out in LA for 6 weeks. That was a lot of fun. We actually took a day trip down to San Diego, so I met a lot of the people who would be my colleagues 8 years later.

HB: Interesting story. When you told me your sister was a psycholinguist, I had assumed that the arrows of causality were working in a somewhat different way. But anyway, she was involved at some level.

VF: She basically nudged and opened doors. This is actually something I bring up with students when they're worried about what careers they should go into and what the right career is for them. I'm convinced that that's just the wrong way of framing that issue. Careers have a lot within them that a person can do. When you land in a place, it's not that hard to find a niche that fits with your personality.

HB: And your passion, presumably. That's something that has to happen. You have to have that fit. You've been exploring these sorts of ideas for a long time and it doesn't seem like your passion is abating at all.

VF: Yes. But I suspect that I would have been just as passionate or as interested in all of these things whether I was a psycholinguist or a vision scientist.

HB: But not solenoids.

VF: Not solenoids, that's right. It needs to be something that can combine a few things together. One of the things I really love about doing cognitive science research is that doing an experiment is not just about developing a better measuring device, or being more precise, or some brute-force thing like that. You really have to come up with a clever way to try to ask a question that indirectly hints at what the answer is.

When I used to teach *Introduction to Psychology*, I would spend half of a lecture talking about these really clever experiments done by Saul Sternberg a number of years ago, trying to get across the idea that Sternberg recognized that you could only report four of these letters. Is that because you only got four of the letters, or is that because you got all twelve and could only report four before they disappeared? He had to come up with this really clever procedure because you can't put a microscope on the brain and say, "*Look. There are the four letters right there.*"

Questions for Discussion:

1. How much of a role do you think chance plays in how our careers develop?

2. What does Howard mean, exactly, when he talks about "priming" during the discussion about a word-recognition experiment with the words always in the same order?

3. Should more effort be made at high school to distinguish between those of a scientific disposition who are motivated to study people and those who prefer less personal fields like physics or chemistry?

II. Minimizing Ambiguity

Finding a linguistic drosophila

HB: I'd like to begin talking about your research by highlighting two points that struck me when reading some of your work. The first concerns the necessity of taking a deeper look at what is actually happening during the communication process. I must admit, I took this completely for granted. I just thought, *If I'm having a conversation with you, of course my job is to communicate with you, and **of course** I'm thinking about the best way to say something so that you can understand it.*

I just assumed that my motivation in forming and pronouncing every word that I pronounce is to make sure that you can actually understand it. But what you're saying is that that's actually not true. To me, that's surprising.

VF: Yes, it turns out to be a bit more complicated than that.

HB: The second point which caught my interest involves how we actually measure that sort of thing anyway, how we're able to design experiments that can lead us to these counter-intuitive conclusions.

VF: Right. Perhaps I'll continue with a biographical approach and explain things that way.

What became my major line of research began with my dissertation, as I think it often does for most academics. It all started when I was in a talk. I was sitting in a chair at the edge of the room, and my advisor at the time—a guy named Gary Dell—was sitting in front of me. Someone said something—whether or not it was the speaker,

I can't remember—that made both of us have the same thought at exactly the same time.

There is a particular sentence structure where a speaker can use the word "that". Think of a sentence like, *The teacher knew that you were going to be late for class*, versus, *The teacher knew you were going to be late for class*. Those are two very similar sentences, and if I hadn't alerted you to the fact that one sentence had a "that" and the other didn't, you probably wouldn't even have noticed that those two sentences were different from one another.

What's valuable about the fact that there are these sorts of sentences, is that the word "that" is practically meaningless. It's very inconspicuous, but nonetheless deciding to use it or not involves your brain making a concrete decision: *this* sentence requires a "that", or *this* sentence *won't* have a "that". And that's exactly what we need.

HB: It's a sort of litmus test.

VF: Yes; it's almost like our linguistic fruit fly, our drosophila. If I can figure out what the factors are that compel a speaker to say, or not say, a "that", I'm going to appreciate something about the way that the sentence-construction mechanism works, the part of our brain that's responsible for putting sentences together.

The thought that popped into my head and my advisor's head at the same time was that sentences like the one I gave you earlier, *The teacher knew you were going to be late*, a type of sentence without the "that", actually contains a momentary ambiguity.

For a brief moment it comes across as if it's going to mean something different and be structured differently than it ends up being structured. That's because, if I said, "*The teacher knew you...*", "you" at that point naturally comes across as if it's the direct object of the verb "know".

HB: Right. If the sentence stopped there it would be, "*The teacher knew you*", which is a completely different kettle of fish than the first example.

VF: Exactly. But that's not what happens. What it does is proceed as: *"The teacher knew you were going to be late."* To put this in linguistic terms, "you" isn't the direct object of the verb "know", "you" is now the subject of an upcoming verb, "were".

The absence of the "that" allows that momentary misinterpretation to occur because if you *do* say the "that", this potential momentary misinterpretation is blocked. If I said, *"The teacher knew that you..."*, I couldn't end the sentence there. At that point, "you" has to be the subject of the upcoming verb, and any ambiguity consequently disappears.

So the thought that occurred to my advisor and me was, *Maybe that's why speakers say "that"?* If we can test this hypothesis, if we can give speakers sentences where, in one case, it will be ambiguous without the "that", while in the other case it will be unambiguous even without the "that", the prediction is that the speaker will be more likely to say the "that" in sentences where it can serve as a disambiguator.

HB: So let me try to summarize a moment. My impression is that when I'm talking to you, I'm trying to be as clear as possible and communicate things as unambiguously as possible.

As the speaker, I'm thinking, *Oh, my goodness, there's potential ambiguity coming. I'm going to ensure that this phrase has maximum clarity because I know that Vic is on the receiving end and he's going to be trying to parse what I'm saying and I'd better make it as easy as possible for him.*

That all makes complete sense, and that's exactly what I thought I was doing all the time whenever I spoke.

VF: That's what I thought was going to happen too and that's what my advisor thought. But we said, *"Let's do this experiment and see."*

So the contrast was between *The teacher knew you were going to be late* and *The teacher knew I was going to be late*, where the key difference between those two sentences lies in the pronoun "you" versus "I". "You" happens to be ambiguous between a direct object role and subject role, whereas "I" is not. "I" has to be a subject.

What we therefore expected to happen is that people would more often insert a "that" in the first sentence—*The teacher knew that you were going to be late*—rather than the second one, because in the first sentence the "that" would serve as a disambiguator, whereas in the second sentence such added disambiguation would be unnecessary.

After all, if that's why speakers say "that"—to block the possibility of a misinterpretation on the part of the listener—then I should say, "*The teacher knew **that** you...*" but I shouldn't bother to say, "*The teacher knew **that** I...*" because that phrase is already unambiguous without the "that".

So what happened? Well, we did three experiments that we were sure were going to demonstrate this effect, but none of them did. The level of "that" usage in a bunch of sentences that had "you" in them, versus a bunch of sentences that had "I" in them, was within 2% of one another, over and over again.

Even with 96 subjects and 48 sentences each—which is a very powerful experiment, if there is a difference to be found, you can usually find it with that much data—it was not there. So we asked ourselves, *What's going on here?*

Along the way, we had done another experiment where we manipulated whether the first subject of the sentence and the second subject of the sentence were the same or different. It was still about "I" versus "you", because we were still testing this ambiguity idea.

This time we used sentences like, *I knew I was going to miss the flight, You knew you were going to miss your flight, You knew I was going to miss the flight*, and *I knew you were going to miss the flight*.

For linguistic reasons, only one of those four—the last one—is potentially ambiguous. The theory that claims that speakers will say "that" to make their sentences as easy as possible for the listener to understand predicts you should say "that" most frequently in this potentially ambiguous sentence. But that's not what happened.

What ended up happening was, for the two sentences that repeat their pronouns—*I knew that I...* and *You knew that you...*—, speakers said "that" significantly less often compared to phrases where the pronouns differed, i.e. *I knew that you...* and *You knew that I...*

That led us to the idea that speakers aren't trying to fashion their sentences, generally speaking, to make those sentences as easy as possible for their listeners to understand after all.

What could be a difference between *I knew that I...* and *You knew that I...*?

Well, when the pronouns repeat, that second pronoun is actually going to be easier for you to think of and say aloud, because it's the same word that you just said a couple of words earlier. But when you consider *You knew that I...*, that second pronoun, "I", is going to be harder to retrieve because it's not a repetition: it's referring to something different.

Questions for Discussion:

1. What does Victor mean, exactly, by the expression "linguistic drosophila"?

2. To what extent does this chapter illustrate the need to rigorously test hypotheses that we suspect are true? How, if at all, does this notion fit into the distinction between "incremental" and "revolutionary" science?

III. Retrieval

Towards objective measurements

HB: Let me ask you a question about practical details. I understand that you have expectations of people using "that" in a particular phrase, or not using "that" in a particular phrase, based upon whether or not it would be appropriate for maximally transmitting clarity from the speaker to the listener.

But how are you getting these people to actually say "that" or not? How does that actually work in practice during the experiment?

VF: This turns out to be one of the things that I actually find to be a lot of fun about the specific area that I study, language production: how is it that people form sentences and convey their intentions accurately?

You have to try to figure out a way to compel people to say the kinds of sentences that you need in order to ask the specific questions that you're asking.

If you're trying to get them to say sentences where the word after the "that" is "I" versus "you", how do you do that, exactly? For that experiment, it turns out that it was safe to rely on the fact that people actually have quite a poor memory for exactly how a sentence is phrased. If you say a sentence to somebody and ask her to say that sentence back to you, she'll remember quite well the gist of the sentence, but often won't remember exactly what particular words were used.

HB: Would you wait any time, or would you just say it to people and then have them say it right back to you immediately? How would that work?

VF: You actually have to break up what we call verbatim memory, or a natural sort of perceptual form of memory. What happened in these experiments was that speakers would see three sentences on the screen. One of them is the one that we care about, and the other two are just filler sentences that I made up. The subjects would read those three sentences one at a time. Then we would take them away. Then I would show them the first few words of one of the three sentences, in random order, so they couldn't anticipate which one they'd get, and then they'd say the sentence back.

So you might read, *The teacher knew that you were going to be late for class*, before reading two other sentences. Then, later on you'd see *The teacher...* and you'd be asked to say that whole sentence back. People's memory for the "that" in this instance is quite poor: it's about 65% or 70% accurate. It's above chance, so they will say it more when it was there and less when it was not, but that ends up being what we call a main effect.

So, overall, people will say the "that" more when it was there and they'll leave it out when it wasn't there, but they do that equally in all of the interesting experimental conditions. If the memory for the "that" isn't interacting with, or isn't related to the other factors that we're interested in, then we can say it's a separate, independent influence, which basically means that we can partial it out.

In those experiments, we just gave people the sentences to read, took the sentences away, asked them to say them back to us, and measured whether they said the "that" or not in those sentences.

As I said, they appear to pay no attention to the potential ambiguity of the sentence. When they are going to say the sentence back, they say the "that" equally, regardless of whether the sentence is going to be ambiguous or not. What they seem to be sensitive to is how easy or hard it is to retrieve the word after the "that". When the word is easy to retrieve, they tend to leave the "that" out. When the word is hard to retrieve, they tend to mention the "that".

HB: And by "retrieving", what do you mean, exactly? What do you imagine is happening in the brain during this process?

VF: The way we envision the sentence production process as working is, basically, that you begin with some notion, what we call a message of the idea that you want to convey.

Then you go through a process of what we sometimes call grammatical encoding, which is retrieving the linguistic features that you think can convey that message—determining the correct words, the correct sentence structure, the proper sounds to be sounded out—which can be shuffled off to articulators so that you can move your lips and create a sound wave that someone else can have impinge on his eardrums and can interpret as a sentence.

In this context, it's a matter of retrieving the individual words to convey the message that we planted in people's heads by having them initially read the sentence.

Again, we believe that the repetition experiment illustrates the fact that what we call *coreferential pronouns*—those that are repeated in the sentence—are easier to retrieve, which compels speakers, more often than not, to leave the "that" out in these cases.

HB: Since they've already used "I" once before, in a sense they're mentally primed to say "I" again.

VF: That's basically the idea.

Another analogy, to give you a sense of ease versus difficulty of retrieval, is to point to situations where we have massive difficulty of retrieval, like when you have a word on the tip of your tongue. If I were to ask you, "*Who was your 11th-grade physics teacher?*" you might think, *Oh gosh, umm...*

You'll know that you know it. If I suggest names, you'll know those are incorrect. That's a situation where retrieval has become so difficult that you actually have to stop what you're doing. That's an extreme case, but one of the things we know is that these things vary on a continuum. Words like "the" and "cat" are very easy to retrieve, while words like "sextant" and "umbrella" are relatively more difficult to retrieve.

HB: Unless you're a mariner.

VF: Yes, unless you're a mariner. Or it rains a lot. Or maybe both.

Questions for Discussion:

1. How might our capacity for retrieval of specific words be dependent on our particular experiences and/or cultural context?

2. To what extent might our capacity for retrieval of specific words or phrases change over time? What might be the causes responsible for such an evolution?

3. Can you see applications of this type of work to Alzheimer's research?

IV. The Division of Labour

Examining message formulation

HB: There's another one of your experiments that I read about that is related to this idea of retrieval. You were asking people to repeat back "writer", "author" in sentences (three words that were roughly synonymous), together with another word like "golfer".

And what you found was that the different word (i.e. here "golfer") was easier to retrieve than the others during this exercise. It seems to me that roughly the same sorts of processes are involved.

VF: Yes. In fact, that's the most direct demonstration of this effect—the ease of retrieval on the mention of the "that". That experiment took advantage of a phenomenon that we've known about in experimental psychology since the 1960s called *proactive interference*. In this case, proactive interference refers to when you find it more and more difficult to retrieve, to remember, words that are similar in meaning to previous words.

The idea is that if you have to remember a list of words that includes "writer", "author", 'poet', 'biographer', by the time you get to 'biographer', you're thinking, *Okay, another writing person, not "writer", not 'poet'; I've already said those things.* The fourth thing suffers from what some people call *cue saturation*: the retrieval cue 'people who write' gets saturated and makes it harder to retrieve that last word.

What you are referring to was an experiment I did with an undergraduate student named Carla Firato. We had speakers say sentences like, "*The writer, the poet, and the author felt that the biographer was boring*" or "*The writer, the poet, and the author felt that the golfer was boring*".

The idea is that "golfer" is easier to retrieve in the context of "writer", "poet", and "author", because it stands out, it doesn't have those same cues. What the experiment showed is a systematic difference, that speakers were less likely to say the "that" with "golfer"—the easier one to retrieve—than with "writer", the one that's more difficult to retrieve.

HB: In the paper, you talk about how you use "that" as a *syntactic pause*.

VF: Yes.

HB: Again, my understanding is that it's related to this notion that I, as a speaker, am thinking, *Okay, I've got this information, but what is that word again?*

So I'll put the "that" in there as I'm searching my mind to come up with the phrase or word that I want to use. I'm not doing this because I predicted, or because I even care perhaps, what you're taking away from this conversation. I'm doing it because I have something to say and I can't say it very quickly, because I have to think about it.

So it seems to me that all of these experiments that you're doing are building towards this conclusion that, when we're having a verbal exchange, the speaker is more fixated on himself and speaking, rather than being concerned about the listener's comprehension—which, again, is very counterintuitive.

VF: That's basically where this whole line of research got off the ground. The initial insight that my advisor and I had—which proved to be wrong—that speakers would say the "that" to make their sentences unambiguous, is based on this intuition that you were just describing.

We feel as though our job as speakers is to construct sentences that are as easy as possible for the listener to understand. So if I have a choice between one that's easier or more difficult for my listener to comprehend, the system presumably was designed, or has evolved, to choose the easier one, thereby making me better at my job of having the listener understand me. But, in fact, that's not the case.

As it turns out, ambiguity and difficulty for the speaker are probably largely independent of one another. It's not that I actually *aim* for things that are potentially ambiguous because that will be easier for me, it's that I'm not paying attention to certain forms of ambiguity when I'm trying to choose whether to say a "that" or not, or whether to put a certain, what we call prosody, on my sentence: where I lengthen certain phrases or shorten certain phrases because that could serve a disambiguating function.

For example, if I say, "*While the man drank, water fell on the floor,*" that big pause between "drank" and "water" indicates that you shouldn't think the water is what's being drunk.

It's easy to overstate it, so let me characterize the big picture of what ends up being called the division of labour. The intuition we have is that, as a speaker, my job is to construct a sentence such that my ideas can be understood as easily and efficiently as possible.

Ambiguity is something that blocks easy comprehension, so we should avoid it too, if possible. The reason that our original intuition, according to this framework, is perhaps incorrect, is because it turns out that, as a speaker, I've got a pretty big job to do all on my own.

As a speaker, every time I formulate a sentence I have to come up with the message that I want to get across. We call that message formulation. I have to search my vocabulary—which has between 30,000 and 80,000 words, depending on exactly what you count as a word—for just those words that will work. If you pull out a dictionary that has 30,000 words, it's a couple of inches thick, so just imagine searching that for the seven words that you want; it's a very efficient process, but nonetheless, from a computational perspective, it's a difficult one. I have to figure out the correct grammatical ordering of those words so that I convey who's doing what to whom, and it's a valid grammatical structure in my language. I have to figure out how to sound out the words. And I have to figure out how to impose the right prosody on the sentence. All this at a rate of about two to three words per second, so 300 milliseconds per word.

HB: There's a lot going on.

VF: Absolutely: there's a lot going on. And then to additionally say, *"And the system should evaluate whether an alternative that you haven't formulated is easier to understand than the one that you're about to formulate,"* requires the system to represent both the utterance you're formulating and that alternative that you weren't even formulating, do the comparison of those two utterances in terms of a process you're not engaging in—namely, understanding the utterances—and choose the easier one.

When you formulate the computational problem that way, I think it goes some way towards illustrating the difficulty of trying to perform additional tasks.

HB: In other words, just in terms of processing power, there are all these constraints involved in my task of forming an appropriate utterance. And if I look at the whole system, there are so many constraints and so many problems to solve, and I only have so much processing power and so much time to be able to do it. So this is the best way to focus on doing things correctly, given the system.

VF: That's basically the idea. In addition to processing power, time pressure, etc., to burden the speaker also with attempting to craft these utterances that are optimally efficient to comprehend—if I can put it that way—is putting too much of a burden on that system in terms of what it's capable of doing.

Questions for Discussion:

1. Do you think it's appropriate for Victor and Howard to be using expressions like "processing power" and "computational problem" to describe how humans speak? Do you think that scientists in the 19th century would speak that way when describing similar experiments?

2. How would you describe, in your own words, what Victor means by "the division of labour"?

V. Disambiguating Ambiguity

Linguistic vs. conceptual

VF: But—and this is where a little more nuance is necessary—it turns out that, generally speaking, we actually do avoid ambiguity really well.

HB: How does that happen?

VF: The argument is something like this: there are different types of ambiguity. One type of ambiguity is what you might call grammatical ambiguity, which is ambiguity that arises because something about the linguistic features of your utterance lend that utterance to mean more than one thing.

HB: Like that famous Groucho Marx joke: *"I shot an elephant in my pyjamas..."*

VF: *"...what he was doing in my pyjamas, I'll never understand."* That's right.

So that ambiguity simply arises because the phrase *"in my pyjamas"* can attach—that's the linguistic lingo—in two different places in the sentence.

I don't need to go into the linguistics of it, but the only way we figure out the syntactic structure of a sentence is by inferring it from the order of words. And in that case the order of the words doesn't strictly determine whether it attaches low or attaches high. That's a linguistic ambiguity because it has entirely to do with this particular set of linguistic features, those words in that order, lending them-selves to two alternative interpretations.

But a different form of important ambiguity that we are very sensitive to is what we sometimes call non-linguistic ambiguity or conceptual ambiguity. This is where you have two things that can be described with the same label because they're very similar sorts of things, or the same thing.

For example, right now, in this room, there are three lights. If there was an issue with one of them, you couldn't just say, "*Deal with that light,*" without doing something to disambiguate which light you were talking about.

It turns out that in that case we're great. There was a set of experiments that I did with my former student Bob Slevc and research assistant at that time, Erin Rogers, where we showed people a display of pictures that had some target object that we were interested in.

We wanted to see how our subjects would describe the target, a critical foil object, and two filler objects that just made things a little more complicated. The target object would be a bat—the flying animal—and the critical foil object in one condition was another sort of bat, a baseball bat.

In another case, it was another bat of the flying type, so then there would be a larger flying bat and a smaller flying bat.

And then in a third condition, we inserted something that was completely unrelated, so that was sort of a control to see what people call this thing in a baseline case.

We told our subjects, "*Describe the thing that we're indicating in a way that someone who's looking at this display could know which of the four objects that you're talking about.*"

So if there was a larger flying bat and a smaller flying bat just calling one of them "bat" wouldn't work because you wouldn't know which one it was. When that's the case, when there is a larger flying bat and a smaller flying bat, people are very clear. They almost never just call them "bat"; they always call it "large bat" or "small bat".

But when it's a flying bat and a baseball bat, they are not nearly as good. They find that to be a much more difficult task: to recognize that if they call this thing "bat", their listener isn't going to know that they're not referring to this other thing over here that's also a bat.

So that, we argue in this paper, illustrates an important distinction between linguistic ambiguity—flying bat versus baseball bat is a linguistic ambiguity because it's just an accident that these two different meanings happen to get mapped onto the same word in English.

That type of ambiguity we're not very good at avoiding, because it requires us to do additional processing: it basically takes up too much computational effort to determine this alternative meaning that you're not intending to use, that you haven't thought of at the moment; and that could be a threat of ambiguity. But when it's a large bat and a small bat, because the two things are similar to each other in meaning, that's actually something we're very sensitive to.

HB: So what's going on? Why do you suspect that people are sensitive to this ambiguity in one case and not the other?

VF: The idea is that all of this has to do with the way that the processing system works and unfolds.

As I mentioned, the general overall framework that most people in my field work with is that you start with this message, you retrieve linguistic features, and then you sound it out. The process of formulating the message is all about what the individual features of meaning are that I need to use to have my intention successfully realized.

If my intention is to describe one thing so that I can distinguish it from another thing, I'm doing that at the level of picking the meaning I'm trying to get across. Small bats and large bats are similar to one another in meaning; and that similarity is something that the system can use to say, "*Oh, there's the threat of ambiguity here; there's a threat that the person is not going to know what I'm trying to get across, so I need to add additional information.*" All of this is happening at this initial level of deciding what the meaning is of what you're going to say, rather than what the words are that you're going to use.

The process of going from the meaning to the words is where the system becomes blind to additional features, because the idea is that the system is thinking, *This is the meaning I want to get across. It's this type of flying mammal. The word 'bat' does that job.* At the level of meaning, you're not able to diagnose the similarity that causes ambiguity because the flying bat and the baseball bat aren't similar to one another in meaning, so you don't, at that stage, formulate the additional features that you need to distinguish the two, because the absence of similarity at that level doesn't let the system recognize that this is going to be a problem. So you just chose the word "bat" once you get to the linguistic level.

Questions for Discussion:

1. What, exactly, does it mean to start with a "message", if the core contents of that message don't explicitly involve words to start with?

2. To what extent do the results of Victor's "bat experiment" argue for a fixed ordering of brain processes involved in speech? How might this be tested further?

3. Do you think that some languages naturally involve a higher frequency of linguistic ambiguity than others? If so, how would you expect native speakers of such languages to fare on these tests compared to speakers of languages with a smaller amount of linguistic ambiguity?

VI. Probing with Pronouns

A future experiment

VF: Here's an experiment that I've never done, but I've always wanted to do. I just haven't had the right people with the right expertise available to me. So if anybody reads this and wants to do this experiment, I'd love it if they would.

One of the ways that we seem to avoid ambiguous utterances in language is with pronouns. Pronouns have a terrible threat of ambiguity because, in English for example, they basically convey two things: what gender something is—"he" or "she"—and whether something is animate or inanimate, because you can also use "it" for an inanimate object.

One of the things we know from other experiments that have been done, is that an English speaker will actually avoid using a pronoun when there's a threat of ambiguity due to the referents being of the same gender. So if I do an experiment—these experiments have typically been done with Disney characters for whatever reason—where Donald and Mickey are going down a hill and then Donald is going to do something after that, I would show the test subject the first picture of Donald and Mickey, ask her to describe what's going on, and then show her the second picture of Donald doing something else afterwards and ask her to again describe what's going on. Then I would repeat the same experiment, but using pictures of Donald and Daisy.

In the first situation with Donald and Mickey, when people describe what's going on with Donald in the second situation, they will use "he" relatively less often, because "he" could refer to either Donald or Mickey. If it's Donald and Daisy, they will use "he" more often to refer to Donald because "he" can't refer to Daisy.

You might think, Well, people don't want to use "he" in the first case with Donald and Mickey because you wouldn't know exactly who was being referred to. And to that I would say, "*Yes, that's what's going on, but the reason the system is able to do that is because Donald and Mickey are similar in the relevant feature of meaning; namely they're both male.*"

The thing that causes the ambiguity is something that's available at the level of meaning and not just at the level of the words you use. Whereas, in the case of Donald and Daisy, they're more different in meaning, so that cues the system that a pronoun is potentially sufficient.

How would you test this idea? What you'd want to do is look at a language that has grammatical gender, that assigns gender to things that are inanimate.

I don't know any of these languages, which is why I haven't been able to do the experiment. In some languages when you refer to things by pronouns, you have to use a pronoun that includes the grammatical gender of the item.

The argument is that, if you did an analogous experiment, where you had two objects and you had to refer to one of those objects, and they had the same grammatical gender, versus having different grammatical genders—so a table and a desk chair perhaps have the same grammatical gender, and a table and an armchair have different grammatical genders—you wouldn't get a difference in pronoun usage between table versus desk chair and table versus armchair, because it's not about the meaning of those things. It's just a quirk of language that one gets male and one gets female.

So the system at the level of meaning doesn't have access to the information that tells the system these things are too similar to one another.

HB: So the idea is to use this to explicitly probe the difference between the meaning aspect from the grammatical aspect?

VF: Yes, the intention is to determine whether this is a meaning-level effect or a grammatical-level effect.

The sort of framework that I've been pushing over the years suggests that whenever some aspect of what I'm trying to get across refers to a difference at the level of grammar, that's kind of a black box that the system, once it starts with the meaning, goes into and just tries to construct the grammar as efficiently as possible and no longer pays attention to what the listener might need.

The work to figure out what the listener might need happened at the first step. So this grammatical gender versus biological gender experiment is a way of trying to tease those aspects apart, because biological gender is at the level of meaning and grammatical gender is at the level of linguistic features.

Question for Discussion:

1. How would you use the examples of large flying bat, small flying bat and baseball bat invoked by Victor in Chapter V to describe the experiment suggested in this chapter?

VII. Grammar

Examining its function

HB: I want to talk a little bit about grammar as a whole, as a concept. You mentioned how the rules of grammar act as a conduit for some quantity of basic information to pass from the speaker to the listener. In your view, as I understand it, grammar is a black box that imposes some structure on me to express myself in a particular way. Perhaps I could look at grammar as a black box with an arrow or something— as a mechanism, basically, through which this information transfer is happening. Is that a fair way to look at it?

VF: Yes.

HB: But of course the rules of grammar are different in different places, and language is different in different places. How much of this actually has to do with languages and cultures in which people find themselves immersed, and how much is something standard that would apply to humans as a whole? Should we be able to see, more or less, these sorts of effects in different people independent of what particular language they speak?

VF: According to this framework, this should be universally true. There are, of course, profound differences in cultures with respect to communicative practices. There are profound differences in individuals across different languages in terms of how they do what they do grammatically. This framework suggests that, given what a grammar does for a speaker, the differences that we see across different languages should be explainable, in part, in terms of trying to satisfy the constraints that are operating.

Let's see if I can give an example of this. Earlier on, you asked, *"If I, as a speaker, am relatively oblivious to the potential ambiguity of my utterances, how do we end up communicating with one another? How do I avoid ambiguity at all?"*

Part of the answer to that question at the grammatical level is that you don't really pay attention to ambiguity, so you're not really avoiding it. How come communication doesn't break down at that point? That's where, as you just mentioned, the grammar steps in.

I should say first of all, that the word "grammar" can mean different things. In this context, what I'm referring to is the set of conventions that determine that certain sentences in my language are permissible and other sentences are not, or that imposing prosody in one way sounds normal and is something I would do, but in other ways sounds unnatural and is not something I would do.

So we have a set of rules—soft rules—in our head that basically tell us, *If this is the type of meaning that you want to get across then these are the grammatical options you have available to you.* Then eventually, when you spit it out, you're going to have to use these words with a preposition of a certain type, or whatever.

The claim is that this grammar is probably shaped—this is speculative on my part—by the language acquisition process, by how it is that we learn languages when we're kids and we pick up on certain features of the language. It's shaped so that ambiguities that exist are tolerable, in terms of eventually getting your ideas across.

Here's the example that I use to try to illustrate this, which takes advantage of cross-linguistic differences. Generally speaking, there are two sorts of languages in the world—it's actually a continuum, but it's good to talk about it as if it's a categorical distinction.

There are fixed word order languages (English is one of those) and there are what are called free word order languages. Japanese is an example of a free word order language. In a fixed word order language, the subject and object of the sentence are determined pretty much entirely by the order of the words in a sentence. So if I say, *"The cat chased the dog,"* you know who's doing the chasing and who's being chased, because "the cat" precedes the verb and "the dog" follows the verb.

But languages like Japanese don't work that way. What they do is they have these things called case markers: little suffixes that you plunk at the ends of words that tell you what the role of that word is in a sentence. In Japanese, then, you wouldn't say, "*The cat chased the dog.*" You would say—I don't know Japanese so I'll have to give you a sort of mixed version—something like, "Cat-ga dog-o chase."

The verb goes at the end, while "ga" tells you the cat is the chaser, and "o" tells you that the dog is the one being chased. Because these suffixes tell you what the subject is and what the object is, you're not constrained to saying, "cat-ga dog-o chase"; you can say, "dog-o cat-ga chase" and it still means "*the cat chased the dog*". And Japanese speakers do that; it's called "scrambling".

So these two types of languages (again, these things are actually on a continuum) work in these two different ways. It turns out that these things tend to trade off against one another. Fixed word order languages like English don't have these suffixes that tell you what the subject and object is. Free word order languages, like Japanese, tend to have these suffixes that tell you what the subject is and what the object is.

What you don't get—very, very rarely, if it happens at all—are languages that are of free word order without case markers. So you wouldn't have a language where you can say "cat dog chase" or you can say "dog cat chase" and those things both mean, "The cat chased the dog." Why doesn't such a language exist? Because it would be intolerably ambiguous. If I could say "cat dog chase" and it could mean either thing, then I can't convey the idea that I'm trying to get across.

So within this framework, the idea is that the grammar ends up allowing a speaker—or enforcing, if you will—options on speakers that will allow them the choices that will generally get across the idea that they're trying to get across.

As I've already mentioned, an example of this in English is that the word "that" is optional in lots of sentences.

There are different kinds of "that"s which are optional. But there's one type of "that" that's not optional, which is a "that" before what's called a subject relative clause. As we've already discussed, you can say, *The man I liked went skiing* or you can say, *The man that I liked went skiing*. These are objective relative clauses, and both versions are grammatically correct.

On the other hand, a subject relative clause would be something like, *The man that liked me went skiing*. You can decide to omit the "that" here and say, *The man liked me went skiing*. In this case, the "that" is not optional.

Why is it the case that the word "that" is not optional in this last case? One possible explanation is that if I say, *The man liked me went skiing*, that sounds so much like I'm saying, *The man liked me*, that it ends up not being tolerated by the grammar. If people started saying that, it would be sufficiently communicatively disruptive to regularly drive people to ask, "*Pardon?*" It would eventually get selected out of the grammar.

Questions for Discussion:

1. Might we be able to use the linguistic distinctions described in this chapter to quantitatively assess which languages are objectively harder to master for native speakers of certain other languages?

2. Why do you think that speakers of free word order languages like Japanese would sometimes opt to "scramble" their sentences?

VIII. Monitoring

Speaking carefully

HB: I'd like to ask you a somewhat different question now. You have this theory about what's happening with most of us when we're speaking. Now you've got me thinking, *Okay, these people aren't actually paying attention to whether their interlocutors are bothering to understand: they're just talking away, grammar is basically taking care of things, while the guys on the other side might have to do some work to properly parse the words to discover the actual intended meaning.*

So you've convinced me that that's what's usually happening when people talk to each other. But now let's look at some special cases: when I listen to people who are very well-trained public speakers, it seems to me that they're being very, very deliberate in the way that they're using language. In particular, my sense is that they are thinking very clearly and effortfully about how they are communicating their ideas. Or take a poet: here is someone who deliberately plays with ambiguities, who plays with the structure of the language—again, in a very effortful way. I'll grant you, it's not something that happens automatically, but it is perhaps what might be called a higher-level function.

Let me be even more personal for a moment. I've recently spent quite a bit of time being forced to think in another language. These days I regularly find myself very much thinking about the structure of grammar, how best to convey my message, and what it would be like as the listener to hear what I'm saying: can the listener actually understand the difference when I say *this* as opposed to *that*?

And I've found—I don't know if this is common, but I suspect it probably is—that when I speak English this sort of thing has rubbed off on me as well, so that I'm now thinking somewhat differently in my native tongue: trying to speak a little bit slower and think more carefully about what I'm saying.

Which is all to say that, as we're talking, I find myself feeling somewhat bemused about this whole idea of efficiency and productivity in terms of minimizing the time taken to say something—that as a speaker, I'm anxious about getting my message out there as quickly as possible.

I can see, of course, the evolutionary argument—or evolutionary effect—behind this sense of efficiency and productivity: that we have to get our messages out there quickly to make sure that a big woolly mammoth doesn't come and eat us while we're struggling to express ourselves.

But in a civilized society where people are trained and cultivated to be high-level thinkers and hopefully develop a reasonably penetrating vocabulary, be sufficiently able—and, moreover, willing— to distinguish between shades of grey, and so forth, it seems a bit different. After all, surely an essential part of what we mean by cultivation and education is actually *transcending* these sorts of constraints?

So that's my confusion. Maybe your conclusions are universal, but in some ways I'm wondering if this isn't just another way of describing a bar that should be crossed. Maybe we should interpret these sorts of results by recognizing that part of being a civilized, cultivated individual is to actually go *beyond* these large-scale constraints and tendencies. Do you see where I'm going here? Does this make any sense at all to you?

VF: It does. I think there might be a couple of ways to bring these two ideas together, both what you're trying to get across and the sort of approach that my colleagues and I have been using in this area.

When you speak of the poet playing with language and ambiguity—that's something you can really use effectively in certain creative forms of communication. And not just poets: think of an administrator who is trying to convey a message to somebody—

HB: There is so rarely an overlap between poets and administrators.

VF: That's exactly right. I chose the other end of the continuum. But if you've ever needed to craft an email very carefully because it's regarding some very sensitive subject, what you do—and I assume a poet is routinely doing the same sort of thing—is to try out the options. You'll write a sentence or a paragraph and then you'll reread it and reread it and make sure it's getting across what you need to get across—no more and no less. And sometimes you'll take advantage of ambiguity to make sure you don't convey something that you feel ought not be conveyed.

That illustrates another component to this process, which, going back to the cognitive psychology of it, we call monitoring. Monitoring is an aspect of language behaviour that you can think of as hearing that voice in your head saying what you're going to say before you actually say it aloud. There's good evidence that we do, in fact, monitor our speech and we can catch it just before it comes out of our mouth—at least if we're not under some big time pressure. When you're giving a talk or a speech this is very hard to do, because you're worried about lots of other things. But during a normal conversation this is something that happens.

The evidence for this comes from a really clever experiment that was done in the 1970s. My field, the study of language production, got off the ground mainly through the study of speech errors. How do we figure out how this system is working when we can't force people to say certain things? These geniuses in the 70s, a woman named Vicki Fromkin (who passed away a number of years ago), Merrill Garrett, and a few other people, recognized that when people make speech errors there's a lot of systematicity in what's going on.

One type of speech error that people make was made famous, perhaps intentionally, by the Reverend Spooner, which we call spoonerisms. Basically, it's when you swap the initial sounds of two words in an utterance and say things like, "The queer old dean" instead of the "The dear old queen," or, "You hissed my mystery lecture," instead of, "You missed my history lecture." Spoonerisms now play a role in our field. People do this unintentionally all the time. A lot of people were suspicious that Reverend Spooner was doing this on purpose, at least sometimes.

Bernie Baars, Michael Motley, and Don MacKay did these experiments in the 70s. You can elicit these spoonerisms by using a priming technique where you give people pairs of words, and then they get a critical word, and the pattern in the previous words makes it so that they might swap the two sounds and create a spoonerism.

What they did was they had people say these phrases where they could end up eliciting a socially inappropriate expression. For example, a relatively notorious one is "Hit shed." If you spoonerize that, you end up with a phrase that's not used in polite company.

So now you can ask the interesting question, *Does the fact that this spoonerism will be socially inappropriate make it any more or less likely that you'll do it?* It turns out that the answer is yes, it does. You are less likely to make a spoonerism that creates something that's socially inappropriate, compared to one that is not.

HB: So there's a check in the system.

VF: There's a check that makes sure. And here's the thing that really clinches the fact that it's something that happens by you hearing it in your head before you say it aloud: the other brilliant thing they did was to measure what's called the galvanic skin response, or GSR.

You put sensors on people's skin that basically measures the sweat level in their skin. You sweat more in situations that are a little higher in anxiety. What they showed was that not only are people less likely to produce these spoonerisms that are socially inappropriate; when they don't do it, their galvanic skin response becomes momentarily higher, as if they momentarily constructed the spoonerism and recognized that it was not something they wanted to do: their GSR spiked.

So that's knockdown evidence that we actually *do* formulate our utterances, hear them in our heads before we say them aloud, and then correct them if it's something that's not what we want to say.

As a process, that is a rather brute-force way of getting around everything that I've been saying in this conversation so far. Yes, you have an idea. That idea enters the grammatical black box and tries to pick out the linguistic features that can be used to get the idea across and that gets formulated into an utterance. How I've been talking so far is with regard to a situation where you then just spit that utterance out, but then there's this monitor process that can hear the linguistic form before it comes out of your mouth, and if it thinks that there's something really wrong with the utterance, it will fix it.

I think that's what poets do when they're playing with the sound of language to try to get across something additional to just what the explicit meaning of the words is, or what the contract writer or academic administrator is doing: putting that monitoring process in overdrive. When you're proofreading something, that's just you monitoring your own production behaviour to see if it says what you want it to say.

Whether you could extend that to broad cultural differences—the British, for example, are known for being careful about how they say things—

HB: Some British. The football hooligans are typically not very careful with their use of language.

VF: Yes, that's right. I suppose we could consult other cultural stereotypes to think of countries where people are considered to be more blunt in terms of what they get across.

In cognitive psychology terms, perhaps you could pin that difference on the degree to which this monitoring mechanism is put to use before people say things aloud. There's good evidence that whatever this monitoring process is, it is what we call resource sensitive: when times get tough, it's something that you'll dispense with because you're trying to deal with other things. One claim would be that you monitor less while you're driving and talking. But it would be reasonable to say that certain cultures might place more of a value on things that would allow them to be more careful about exactly the way that phrasing is made.

Questions for Discussion:

1. What might be some cultural factors that would result in a generally increased or decreased level of monitoring throughout the population?

2. Has the speed of your speech patterns changed over your life? Do you find yourself monitoring your utterances differently now from what you've done in the past?

IX. In the Brain

Brain imaging and language

HB: I've had the opportunity to speak with many people in cognitive science who use all sorts of modern diagnostic techniques like fMRI to investigate their theories, and it seems to me that it would be very interesting to be performing many of the sorts of experiments you've been describing while simultaneously scanning their brains with the likes of fMRI. Have you thought of, or have you already been involved in, fMRI testing to get a clear sense of where in the brain many of these processes are actually happening?

VF: Yes. I recently spent two months in New York City at NYU working with a woman there named Liina Pylkkänen. She uses a different brain-monitoring technique, something called MEG, which stands for magnetoencephalography. It measures the actual magnetic field that's given off by the brain moment to moment. Some time after that I spent two months in Boston at MIT working with a woman named Evelina (Ev) Fedorenko who uses fMRI to study brain activity. In both cases we set up projects that are ongoing.

It's really clear at this point that the fields of behavioural science, broadly speaking, and cognitive science specifically, are going through a kind of a neural revolution. The degree to which neuroscientific techniques are going to be important for doing investigations of cognitive functions is increasing, and it's just going to become more and more important. However, there's a real challenge with using fMRI for the types of questions that we ask.

I think fMRI has been very successful in many areas. One area, for example, is basic perceptual processing, like visual processing. People have used fMRI in humans to understand the way that visual areas work in the back of your brain, doing the sorts of experiments that were simply not available before the advent of fMRI. I have a colleague named Adam Aron who studies the control system in the brain. This is something that inhibits some behaviour that you ought not to do, like if you're walking across the street and suddenly see a car bearing down on you and you suddenly stop your walking behaviour. There's a system in your brain that's responsible for that, and he's been using fMRI very successfully to get a foothold on how it works.

The way that language works in the brain has a couple of features to it that make using fMRI challenging, in my view. One is that it's complex and multifaceted. Language involves meaning, grammatical form, sound, pragmatics—reasoning about what other people think and how they think—and so on. For any given act of language, trying to isolate each of those things is going to be difficult. If they are done in different ways by the brain, that's going to make it very challenging to potentially figure out exactly what is going on with regard to some specific question.

For example, is there a part of the brain that's sensitive to ambiguity? Well, you're going to have to be able to take into account the fact that all these other possible systems might also be relevant to the question you're asking.

The second reason I think it's going to be tough to study language using techniques like fMRI is because of what we call neuroplasticity.

One of the things we know about the brain is that the way psychological functions map onto brain functions can differ from individual to individual. It can also differ within an individual.

If I have a stroke, for example, and suffer some brain damage, my brain will reorganize, to the extent that it can, to recover some of the function that I used to have. One of the things about neuroplasticity is that the brain is relatively less plastic, or less variable, from individual to individual in perceptual areas—like the visual system—and is relatively more plastic in higher-level areas like language and reasoning and so forth. So using fMRI—which basically has the ability to tell you where something is happening in the brain—to study something that might vary a lot from individual to individual, clearly poses a challenge.

HB: And presumably it might also vary over each individual's lifetime as well.

VF: It can certainly vary within an individual over his or her lifetime.

Ev Fedorenko has a way of dealing with at least one of these problems using a technique—developed by a woman she works with named Nancy Kanwisher—which uses what she calls functional localizers. That allows you to at least say, *"What we're going to do, on a subject-by-subject basis, is haul each person into the machine individually. We're going to use some task to measure some function of interest, and then we're going to use other tasks to see whether, for that individual subject, this other task uses the same parts of the brain as the first task."*

In Ev's case, what she's been doing is using a language localizer. She'll give people a bunch of sentences that are grammatical, versus a bunch of gibberish non-word strings; figure out what parts of the brain light up more for the grammatical sentences compared to the gibberish, and then she'll look at some other tasks and see if they rely on the same brain regions.

She and I, along with some other collaborators, are working on a project to use that technique to find out, on a subject by subject basis, what parts of the brain are responsible for language function.

We're studying another thing that we know happens when people produce language. It's called—these things all suffer from jargon—*cumulative semantic interference*.

For example, if I asked you to name a sequence of pictures one after another; and unbeknownst to you these pictures come from a common category—say you name a sheep, and then five pictures later you name a cow, and then seven pictures after that you name a horse—you'll name each successive picture of an animal more slowly than the preceding one. It's a type of learning effect that happens.

Now, using this technique, we can ask the question: is that a language thing, or is that a non-language thing? First we localize the language functions, then we have them do this task, and then we see if it's these language areas or not that light up with this increasing interference effect.

HB: How much variation are you getting in these "language areas" from subject to subject?

VF: A decent amount. Because the other thing that this technique does, which is quite nice, is that it frees you from the need to have a contiguous area that's responsible for a putative psychological function: it's pretty unlikely that there's a single chunk of brain that's entirely responsible for language and nothing else.

By using a technique like this it's free—to the extent of the resolution of the scanner—to find specific areas—we call them voxels—within that region that are for language, whereas a neighbouring voxel might not be sensitive to language.

When you allow that much freedom from one subject to another, potentially no two subjects will be the same in terms of what parts of the brain show language function.

Questions for Discussion:

1. Might it make sense to distinguish between "high level" (like language) and "lower level" neural activity (like perception) to better understand cognitive processing? Why or why not?

2. How do you think the phenomenon of cumulative semantic interference might be explained?

3. Might we one day be able to use fMRI machines to conclusively demonstrate that other animals also use language?

X. Philosophical Divertimento

Brain vs. Mind

HB: A moment ago you mentioned the current neural revolution in cognitive science. It seems to me, as an outsider, that there is one principal, illuminating rift in terms of attitudes of the practitioners of cognitive science. Those of the hard-core neuroscience persuasion seem to believe that there is no fundamental difference between the brain and the mind (i.e. the brain causes the mind and the mind is our own personal subjective manifestation of our brain states), whereas those on the other side of the rift don't subscribe to that.

That isn't to say that they believe the brain has nothing to do with the mind, but they're of the view that there's more to heaven and earth than merely brain states. Typically the first category of people use the word "brain"—they don't even use the word "mind" very much when discussing these issues—while the second category of people use the word "mind". That's my perception of what's going on sociologically, at least.

VF: You've perceived it very well.

HB: Okay. So then my next question is, *Which category of person are you?*

VF: I guess I should just come right out and say that I'm the second category of person, and then hopefully I can explain why I think that's a reasonable stance to take.

My view of people of the second category is that we're all what you would call—I'm going to veer into some philosophical terminology—physicalists. We believe that every mental function is—not just corresponds to, actually *is*—a physical function.

HB: So you're not a Cartesian dualist or anything like that.

VF: Right, I'm certainly not a Cartesian dualist. But I am a *kind* of dualist, what you might call a *functional dualist*. The position is that, even though every mental event is identical to a physical event, the proper characterization of how a behaviour is organized isn't at the level of physical events. If you want to form the categories of mental things and you try to do it at the physical level, you won't be able to do it.

Now, what does that mean, exactly?

Well, what's the physical pattern that corresponds to my conception *dog*? What's the physical pattern that corresponds to *cat* or *mouse*? All of those things are small animals, and so at a level of mental description, if you will, there is a similarity between those three things: that's a category of things. The argument is that, if you had the three physical patterns that correspond to those three mental patterns, there wouldn't necessarily be a physical thing they have in common that corresponds to them being animals.

HB: Okay. Let me back up and be very concrete so that I can understand what you're saying. When you're talking about a physical pattern, I'm assuming that if you said to me, "*Howard, think of a dog*", and I would do so, then there would be something going on in my brain corresponding to that thought, some physical activity—

VF: Presumably electrical interactions among neurons.

HB: Right. And what I think that you're saying is that such a pattern, or brain state, is not the be all and end all of my mental representation of a dog. Or is that not what you're saying?

VF: That's not what I'm saying. It *is* the be all and end all of your mental representation of a dog, but the *physical* characterization, the description of the patterns that correspond to dog in terms of electrical activities—

HB: My brain state.

VF: Yes. Those brain states aren't the way they are to correspond to the relevant mental categories.

Let me try to give you another example of this. It's not sufficient to just talk about dogs to try to get this notion across, you have to talk about things that have some mental organization and things that have some physical organization. The claim is that the mental organization won't necessarily correspond to the physical description or characterization of it.

A little more philosophical lingo might be handy here. Like I said, people on this side of the divide, we all consider ourselves to be physicalists: we all believe that the mind is the brain. But there's an important distinction between what we call *type physicalism* and *token physicalism*.

Type physicalism is the idea that if you have a brain state that corresponds to a particular mental state, then that brain state is in some physical sense the same across individuals and across time. So the brain state that corresponds to *dog* in my head is the same as the brain state that corresponds to *dog* in your head.

HB: And it will be two weeks from now.

VF: Yes, the brain state that corresponds to *dog* in my head will be the same brain state that corresponds to *dog* in my head two weeks from now, in some relevant physical characterization.

Token physicalism, meanwhile, is the idea that, for example, *dog* as a mental state is identical to *dog* as a brain state, but the requirement that this brain state is the same between me and you, the requirement that it's the same for me now as it will be two weeks from now, or ten years from now, does not hold.

HB: Well, I'm sure the hard-core neuroscience guys on the other side of the rift would acknowledge that. The rift seems to have disappeared.

VF: I think they would acknowledge it. I actually had a really interesting discussion about this exact issue in the hallway outside my office about a week and a half ago. They acknowledge it, but I think it's easy to overlook the ramifications of this distinction for how we do cognitive neuroscience.

One way to think about this is in terms of the notion of reduction. Can you reduce a certain type of organization at the mental level to an organization at the physical level? Could you, for example, say, *"Everything that's an animal, in terms of different mental events, corresponds to this particular physical pattern in the brain."*

HB: Well, I think that I implied you could by using the term "brain state". So I was begging the question, at least with the idea of *dog* right?

VF: I don't think you were begging the question, because, like you said, I do think dog represents a brain state—there is nothing other than that.

We can talk about what nouns do in language by drawing a bunch of rules that aren't about neural states or electricity or anything. We can write out "nouns go into noun phrases" and so forth. I firmly believe that every noun that I know in my language corresponds to a brain state in my head. So the question of interest is, *Could I rewrite the rules of language that describe what you can do with nouns in terms of rules of electrical interactions in the brain?* The contention of people like me, on this side of this divide, is that that's not, in principle, possible.

In a sense, it's helpful to think of the causal arrow in the other direction. Most of us, when we think about the fact that the brain is the mind, think that the brain does things and that causes us to have the mental life that we have. But this way of thinking about things, which I've just outlined, suggests that can't be true in any strong sense.

Hopefully during the course of this conversation you've learned some particular fact that you're going to know for some period into the future. That's a mental thing that happened. Somehow that fact that has been learned will cause a series of brain changes that makes it so that is something that ends up being in your head for the longer term.

At some level, unless you think it's all billiard balls, unless you think that what happens when I told you a new fact like, "*I was born in Winnipeg*," is that sound waves impinge your eardrum, cause the three bones to move in a certain way, which then causes the brain to change in a certain way, and it's all happening at the level of the brain—unless you think that it's all deterministic in that way, or you think that it's just stochastic, random, there has to be some sort of mechanism, such that the way you're thinking about something, the function you're trying to accomplish psychologically, can change the way that the brain represents that thing.

I'm not articulating this very well, I'm afraid…

HB: No, I think you're doing fine. But let me now throw aside my cloak of impartiality and declare that I'm in the first camp. Let me take a more concrete analogy because I feel more comfortable when I deal with concrete things. So let me talk about something like the proof of Fermat's Last Theorem.

This involves many complex mathematical ideas and there was this guy named Andrew Wiles who came up with a rigorous proof of this thing, and you are either familiar with that proof or you're not. Now suppose I were to go through it rigorously—which, as it happens, I haven't done and probably couldn't do to any meaningful degree—but I imagine I could do that so that I understand every line of what Wiles had done, then I will have learned something and my brain will have changed, just as it would have changed in some way—presumably another way—had I spent that time learning how to crochet or something.

What's bothering me is the argument in principle, of course, not in practice. So I imagine that I would have one brain state before I sat down to learn about Fermat's Last Theorem, and then I would have a different brain state after learning about Fermat's Last Theorem. The state itself would be horrifically complicated, and I don't think we'll ever be able to quantify it in a gazillion years, but in principle, which is what we're talking about, I would be able to map my brain state before to my brain state afterwards.

And if you can map this brain state completely, which is the supposition—in principle it should be possible to do—if you had a complete understanding of neurophysiological principles, the laws of physics, the laws of chemistry, and all that kind of mysterious stuff (even including the stochastic element that is induced by something like quantum theory), then the claim is that, if you have the initial state, you should be able to predict the final state according to these laws, at least roughly.

VF: Yes, that's right.

HB: So you have these two brain states, and it's all tremendously complicated. But I guess my problem is that, if you believe that, there's nothing else there. However complicated it is, however untenable and unrealistic it is that we would ever be able to meet those assumptions, if you *could* meet those assumptions, then it seems like if you've got one brain state here and another one there, and I understand those principles, then I can say, "*Okay Victor, if you start with this brain state and then you learn about Fermat's Last Theorem, then this will be your brain state afterwards.*" It would be incredibly difficult to extract and we'll probably never be able to; but again, in principle, it's possible. Do you understand what I'm saying?

VF: I do. I think that in the limit it might be possible to do this entirely physically, but to do that you will need to know what would practically be impossible.

HB: Fair enough.

VF: Perhaps still impossible even in a gazillion years, because the idea is this: the physical state of your brain after you've learned Fermat's Last Theorem, versus before, is going to be a function not only of the set of facts that make up the proof of Fermat's Last Theorem, but also all of the other facts that impacted what your brain was like before, the whole context in the middle, the whole context at the end—

HB: Sure. And how good it makes me feel: the meta-stuff. I'm going to feel great because I finally understood this thing, and all of a sudden my brain's going to change because of that too.

VF: And whether or not you had a glass of orange juice is going to affect that set of brain states, and so forth. In principle, because the initial state matters, everything that you did before in your life since, in principle, conception, is going to matter, because the physical state of your brain as you began this process will have been different if ten days before you didn't do some relevant behaviour, compared to something else.

HB: OK, but I'm assuming I can take a snapshot of my brain at a particular time, so to some extent, I don't really care about what I did before. I'm assuming I can set the initial conditions. This is a huge assumption in practice, and I don't think it's going to be possible to ever be able to do, quite frankly. But it's possible *in principle*—that's my argument.

So *if* you could take a snapshot of the brain and could tag everything at one particular time, then I don't care what happened before, what's happened since conception. For the sake of argument, let's say I have a photograph of your brain state at this particular time. That's my claim.

VF: I don't think that's going to work because I think that the way your brain ends up solving the problem of encoding the knowledge that's coming in through your sensory organs could be, in part, affected by what happened before.

I think I know what you're saying. You're saying, "*Well, maybe all of that can actually be captured statically, together with everything that's happening now.*"

HB: And you're saying that probably can't be captured in a snapshot of the brain state at a particular time. Maybe you're right.

So if I were to argue from your perspective, I guess the claim would be that, to understand Fermat's Last Theorem, there doubtless would have been a technique that you would have had to learn at some point in the past and it's not obvious that something like that would necessarily be manifested in the photograph of the brain state. I could imagine two different situations: one person learned this technique and somebody else didn't learn this technique, but just looking at the brain state wouldn't necessarily give you that information. Is that the idea?

VF: That's the position. But now, as you're phrasing it that way, I can see what your position is too.

If you knew every single possible physical state that was relevant, I can see how that would actually allow for all of the previous context to be encoded in that snapshot.

Have we convinced each other of the opposite of our original positions?

HB: Perhaps. I guess the analogue in physics would be some level of what they call degeneracy, right? It's possible to reach one state from a variety of different paths.

VF: That's right. If there's a many-to-one mapping from previous states to this current snapshot—

HB: And you can't disentangle that.

VF: Exactly. That's the possible indeterminacy that would make that true.

Questions for Discussion:

*1. What does Howard mean, exactly, when he says, "**So you're not a Cartesian dualist or anything like that.**" What is "Cartesian dualism" and how is it relevant to this part of the conversation?*

2. If there is no meaningful difference between "the brain" and "the mind" what, if anything, does that imply about free will?

3. Does this chapter make you more, or less, inclined to read a book on the philosophy of mind?

XI. Language and Thought

The Sapir-Whorf hypothesis

HB: Let's return to what we were talking about earlier: this notion that I have a message to convey to you and you're parsing it carefully, trying to understand it, and somehow this big black box of grammar is involved in helping to make sure that the message is decodable, as it were.

Behind all of this there seems to be this assumption that you have two people talking, there is some fundamental message out there, and then we use language to encode that message.

It seems to me there are people who might have a somewhat different perspective. They might say, "*Hang on. It's not as if there is a message or content that we can claim exists independent of language. In fact, language **itself** frames the way we think about the world. We learn about the world **through** language and thus it is **impossible** to imagine a thought or an idea **independent** of language.*" So my first question is, do people actually subscribe to that?

VF: Yes.

HB: And how would you respond to them?

VF: This is a long-standing issue in the language sciences. It's often called the Whorfian hypothesis or the Sapir–Whorf hypothesis, which is an acknowledgement of both people who are credited with first raising this issue.

How Whorf phrased this idea isn't quite as relevant or interesting to talk about as what I think the overall set of issues ends up being. The question is, *What is the relationship between the fact that languages use particular devices to encode thoughts and the way that thought processes are able to unfold and work?*

There's one extreme that I don't think anybody believes—although it has an intuitive appeal—which is the idea that we literally think *in language*: that, if you didn't have language, you wouldn't be able to think at all. That, I think, is patently false. And I think the fact that it's false is illustrated by the fact that, if we thought in language, then we wouldn't ever feel that some linguistic expression of our thought was inadequate. If the only way that I could think was with the words and sentences in my language, all I would need to do is just transcribe that thought into those words and that would be the thought itself.

One of my former advisors, a woman named Kay Bock, would often point out that the fact you have meanings for things that you don't have words for, illustrates this. She would always point to the thing at the end of your shoelace that allows you to thread it through the eyelet. That's a thing, and we know it's a thing, but we don't have a word for it. It's untenable to say that the language that you use to represent that thing is the thing at the end of your shoelace. So I don't think anybody genuinely thinks that we simply think in language.

The other extreme point of view is one that I think a lot of people subscribe to—and I think I subscribe to, but I'm gradually being convinced away from it—which is that throughout all cultures, regardless of the radically different ways that their individual languages might work, everybody is capable of thinking exactly the same way.

One famous way that this debate came out is through differences in what's called a subjunctive construction. A subjunctive construction is something like, "*If it were raining, I'd be carrying an umbrella.*"

It's a way, with one efficient utterance, to describe an implication: *there's an x that implies y: "rain" implies "me carrying an umbrella". But x isn't true: it's not raining.*

Some other languages don't have this. I believe that Chinese, for example, doesn't have a single subjunctive construction. I don't speak Chinese, so I can't verify this first hand, but the claim is that, to express the same thing, you basically have to say something along the lines of, "*If it is raining, then I'd be carrying an umbrella. But it's not raining.*" So you have to explicitly deny the antecedent in a subsequent phrase.

This led to the conjecture that the ability to reason counterfactually might differ between speakers of Chinese and speakers of English, who can phrase, in a simple sentence, a state of affairs that isn't true, but nonetheless, if it were, would have some implication.

So a series of experiments was done to test whether there was any difference in the ability of native speakers of the respective languages to reason counterfactually. But someone else came along afterwards and said, "*It looks like there were some difficulties in how the test materials were translated from the experimenter's language, English, into Chinese.*" My sense of that micro-debate ended up being that there are not strong differences in counterfactual reasoning abilities between English speakers and Chinese speakers. And that, I think, is because, in the limit, a Chinese speaker can simply be more explicit and say, "*If it is raining, then I'd be carrying an umbrella. But it's not raining.*" So when you ultimately need to do the reasoning, you can fall back on other strategies.

HB: Right. But there's a difference between not being able to—which is a very strong claim—and the idea that language increases one's proclivity to think in a particular way. It seems like there's a case to be made for language impinging on one's way of thinking, let alone just expressing thought.

VF: This is often described as what you might call habitual behaviour. It might not be that I *can't* think counterfactually because my language doesn't have the subjunctive, but my *habitual* way of considering things might be influenced by that fact.

HB: Do you believe that's the case, or not?

VF: I'm trying to think what the evidence is on this... One of my colleagues here at UCSD, a woman named Lera Boroditsky who's in the Cognitive Science Department, is more toward the side of this debate that argues that language influences habitual thought patterns. One example that she uses is the fact that different linguistic and cultural communities will describe, for example, the passage of time differently. In English, we describe the future as ahead of us, generally speaking, and we describe the past as behind us. Other cultures do the opposite: they describe the past as in front of you and the future as behind you.

She's done a series of experiments where she argues that this *does* actually strongly affect how you do certain things. She highlights a Nestlé ad campaign some time ago where they showed a series of images of an infant turning into a toddler and then turning into an adult, which went from left to right.

But when it was marketed in Israel, where they read the other way—from right to left—it seemed to suggest that this Nestlé product would actually lead your kid to revert in behaviour.

The fact that we sometimes engage in certain language-related habitual behaviours *does* affect how we interpret things. My sense is that the debate has gone from entertaining quite strong hypotheses that a language not having certain features would prevent you from being able to do certain things, to a strong opposite perspective that says, "*It makes no difference what your language is.*"

And now I think we're converging on the middle position, which is that language can build in certain ways of organizing how you think about time, how you think about events and so forth, that can then affect moment-to-moment behaviours. If the way that you needed to reason about some time process, say, was compatible with the way that your culture tends to use a metaphor for it, then that might make it a little easier for you to reason than if it's incompatible with that. I think the evidence for that is pretty compelling. So it ends up being one of these kinds of middle-of-the-road answers, at least for now.

There is, I think, an analogous situation with the debate over the innate component of language. There's an extreme point of view that says that you're hardwired for language. Noam Chomsky and Steve Pinker represent the point of view that says that your language faculty, to a large extent, is determined by a genetic endowment. One elegant argument on this side—that I suspect isn't true, even though it is quite elegant—is that (going back to a selection metaphor) the features of your language are selected from a finite inventory that is this genetic endowment.

At the other extreme, people argue that language is actually just a highly practiced skill, like chess. If we played chess as much as we used language, we would consider chess to be as remarkable and possibly as innate as many of us now consider language to be.

Again, both of those extremes are probably not true. I think most people who have thought about this would acknowledge that there are innate constraints on the way that language works, but the organizational system is also strongly shaped by learning experiences that occur over your life.

But an interesting aspect of this meta-scientific issue, is that—and this is going to portray folks who take extreme points of view in a favourable light—

HB: Favourable?

VF: Yes. Because you need them. The claim is that—

HB: Oh, I see, methodologically. You need them to set the limits, as it were.

VF: Yes, to set the limits, to represent the extremes. By having people like Noam Chomsky and Steven Pinker on one side, claiming the innate aspect of language, while having, on the other side, people like my late colleague Liz Bates who was a strong proponent of the other side of the argument—that language structure, to a very large extent, is inherited from the environment—*that* allows the debate to be framed in such a way that all of us working in the middle can make progress.

Of course, that only paints them in a favourable light because they're wrong for the sake of framing a debate. But I'm sure they don't see it that way.

Questions for Discussion:

1. What, exactly, does it mean to "reason counterfactually" and how is that relevant to the subjunctive construction Victor mentions?

2. To what extent do you expect you would think differently if you were raised speaking another language?

3. What assumptions lie behind notions like "innate", "natural" and "inherited" when it comes to this debate?

4. Do you think it's fair to represent the views of Chomsky, Pinker and Bates as "extreme"? Why or why not?

XII. Future Investigations

Environmental impacts and big data

HB: You've been very generous with your time, and I'd just like to end with a few more questions. You mentioned some ideas for some possible future experiments earlier on. Where do you see the future of your field more generally?

VF: Where I see a lot of the field going at this point—a number of us are seeing this; this isn't a crystal ball thing—is that a confluence of factors are pushing things in an interesting new direction. This is actually somewhat relevant to this innate versus learned debate on language structure we just mentioned. There are a number of factors pointing us toward a belief that our language knowledge is, in fact, shaped by ongoing experiences in a way that we hadn't quite appreciated before.

There's a whole new line in cognitive science that has risen to prominence in the last 10 or 15 years that views a lot of what human beings do in terms of their behaviour patterns as, in a way, optimal.

The common thread in a lot of this research is to take some instance where a human was seemingly behaving irrationally and show that, in fact, he's behaving rationally when you take into account all the other factors that might be relevant.

In the language sciences this has been unfolding in a way that suggests that the way we understand language, the way that we produce language, isn't just some fixed grammar that gets into our head and stays that way.

Rather, by responding to contingencies in our environment, our language system will change and adapt. This is often framed in terms of what's called a Bayesian framework: the idea that when a language comprehension system, for example, is trying to estimate what a piece of language might mean, it's taking into account all of the prior information that it has, and given that prior information, it tries to figure out what the most likely interpretation of that thing is.

From a production perspective you can imagine a sort of reverse process along those lines. If the system really is optimal in that way, how does it become optimal, given all of the variation across time, a person's language and life, and across different people?

The idea is that you end up having the system be that way because it's quite sensitive to past experience in a way that tweaks it so that it can adjust its prior probabilities.

HB: So this is some sort of an evolutionary argument on some level.

VF: Evolutionary, but not genetic selection, obviously.

HB: Sure.

VF: It's almost a tuning argument. My lab is moving in this direction as well: we're spending more time looking at what are the ways that you can show that there is some learning event that happened in your recent past that's now going to change the way that you end up describing something in the future.

I'm trying to think of a good concrete example. All of this is still in its infancy.

One aspect is this optimal notion, another is the experience-dependent notion of learning—the idea that recent experiences cause changes in the way that you do language, the way you process language.

And a third component is the degree to which this ends up being context-sensitive. With regard to this third component, I can talk about one set of studies that's going on in my lab.

One of the things we do in our field is study situations where there is a given message to express involving two reasonably good alternatives that could be used to do so, such as using a "that" or not.

There are, of course, other versions: you can imagine a card that has a line drawing that shows a man putting beers into a cooler. There will be two people in the room, an experimenter and a subject, and they'll take turns describing cards to one another.

There are 12 cards in front of the experimenter, and each of the cards can be described in one of two ways: for example, *The man is loading beers into a cooler* or *The man is loading the cooler with beers*; *The woman is giving an apple to the teacher* or *The woman is giving the teacher an apple* and so forth for all 12 different cards.

As the experimenter, I describe the first card to you and you find it in your set and put it in the pile. I'll do this for 12 sentences using what we call three different alternations.

The first one is what's called a locative alternation: *The man is loading beers into the cooler* or *The man is loading the cooler with beers*.

The second one is what we call a ditransitive alternation: *The woman is giving the apple to the teacher* or *The woman is giving the teacher the apple*.

And then the third one is likely the most familiar one to people, the transitive—active versus passive: *The alarm clock is waking up the boy* or *The boy is being awakened by the alarm clock*.

So you get 12 of these in a row, which is quite a bit, and now it's the subject's turn to do the same thing. So the subject gets those same 12 pictures and has to describe them back to the experimenter.

HB: So, *Is the subject influenced by what the experimenter says?* Is that the idea?

VF: That ends up being the question: for any given picture does the subject end up using the same structure that the experimenter used?

If we are able to show that, it would be pretty surprising to some extent, because as I said earlier, we have quite poor memory for exactly how a sentence was phrased.

Across the several minutes that it takes the experimenter to describe this entire set of pictures and for the subject to then describe them back, plus the interference of those other 11 sentences being part of the same set, if the subject nonetheless *still* retains enough of that initial description to end up saying it back using the same structure, that would be surprising.

But that is what we find; the subject is about 10% to 20% more likely to use the structure the experimenter used, compared to a new one.

That's kind of interesting. It shows that the subject has picked up on something in the environment: a relationship between some thing that the experimenter described and the structure used to describe it, and the subject then encoded that, which influenced the subject's future production behaviour.

Now the quest is to figure out what this mechanism is sensitive to. Is this something that your brain is doing robustly? If I describe these 12 cards to you and then you go away for a week and you describe the same 12 cards back to me, will you show the same effect? If we do it in a different room will the effect go away?

HB: And what if there are other people around?

VF: Right. Or what if we tweak the colours of the picture slightly?

That makes it sound sort of like a fishing expedition, but the point is to recognize that your behaviour of describing a picture in a particular way is going to be sensitive to a whole set of contextual features, and the extent to which it is or isn't sensitive to a particular feature is probably going to tell us whether the way that your language system is working is somehow optimized. It has recognized that a specific type of contextual feature is relevant, and it's going to take that contextual feature into account.

HB: I suppose that it will be more sensitive to some things and less to others.

VF: Presumably as a function of those things relevant to the learning process, or what it would be good for me to know about how the sentence might come out.

Another important happening in the field right now is, to use a popular phrase, big data. In some ways the language aspect of cognitive science has been able to harness big data more easily than many other areas, because it turns out that there are massive databases of language everywhere.

Newspapers are all available online and we can use them as a database of language. The World Wide Web is a huge database of language, and with the right tools you can now go in and measure to what extent particular, subtle, patterns are actually coming out in these massive databases of language. You can address questions through these very large databases such as, *Do people tend to repeat structures that they've recently heard in some particular context?*

HB: There's a lot of data out there. It's just a question of how you parse it and how you try to isolate various factors that might be responsible for the learning process. That's the problem, I'm guessing.

VF: There are two issues: one is parsing and the other is enriching. A sequence of words in a database doesn't tell you what the structure of that sentence is and what the individual categories are. And it's often in those ways that our hypotheses are phrased. So you need to not only be able to figure out how to pull the pieces of data out, but how, if there is a whole lot of it, you can then tag things so that you've coded the relevant variables that you're interested in.

Questions for Discussion:

1. Can you imagine some other plausible interpretations of the results Victor is getting from the experiment he describes here?

2. Do you sometimes find yourself picking up and repeating the speech mannerisms of other people you are regularly around? If so, how might that be relevant to the concepts discussed in this chapter?

XIII. Mind-Brain Redux

The debate continues...

HB: Anything else I haven't asked that you'd like to talk about? Something you'd like to talk about some more?

VF: I'd actually like to go back to something we were talking about earlier, namely the mind-brain issue.

There was a really interesting talk the other day by this guy from UCLA who was describing a project related to the National Institutes of Mental Health. The project involved looking for the brain basis of different sorts of psychological disorders. The idea is that if we can come up with a good taxonomy of factors that are relevant to psychological disorders and look at what the brain systems are that correlate with the relevant features of these mental disorders, that's going to help us get a foothold on trying to understand these mental disorders and potentially cure them eventually.

One hypothesis is that we can analyze the efficiency of transfer of brain signals from one part of the brain to another, correlate that with these different features of mental disorders, and see the extent to which that can explain—or at least seem to be related to—those features of the disorder.

It was a really interesting talk and a really good idea, but I see it as fundamentally wrong-headed. The analogy that I would use is an age-old one in the cognitive sciences field that is relevant to this rift that we were discussing earlier.

As everyone knows, one of the problems we have with our computers is that they get these disorders called viruses, which cause massive problems with the way they work. If we wanted to cure a computer of a virus, the category-one type of approach would be,

OK, let's go into the physical makeup of the computer and try to find what it is physically about this computer that's causing this problem.

But I'm sceptical that would be a very efficient way to go about doing it, because the nature of the virus is relatively *independent* of the physical factors that correspond to what that virus is. Instead, an effective "computer doctor" would go in, look at the software, try to isolate what this thing is, and try to delete it using some software.

The analogy to the human brain and mental health is clear: if somebody has some condition like ADHD or autism, it's possible that there is a relatively simple, relatively tractable physical thing that we could point to and say, *"This corresponds enough to this mental disorder, so if we deal with this physical part, the mental thing is going to fix itself,"* but it's also possible that it isn't at that level at all. It's possible that, for many of these disorders, the problem is happening at this functional level.

Perhaps an intuitive example of this would be post-traumatic stress disorder, or PTSD. PTSD has some genetic, hardwired component to it—there's a diathesis that leads to it—but then there's a stress event that causes it. That stress event is instrumental in the way that the condition unfolds and plays out: reliving the event, trying to compartmentalize it in certain ways, and so forth.

The analogy to the virus idea would be that trying to figure out what's going on with PTSD by figuring out what the physical thing is that corresponds to this condition might not make as much sense as figuring out what this traumatic event was, how it's being remembered at a psychological or mental level, how it's now playing out in terms of being compartmentalized and being relived so that we can try to isolate it.

If you believe that a digital computer with a hardware and a software level isn't something magical, isn't something with a soul that somehow manages to magically rewire the ones and zeros so that it ends up having the behaviour that it does, then the idea is that the mind is doing the same thing. The way the system is playing out functionally is what ends up having the physical system represented the way that it is.

HB: Let me give a response, as an avowed category-one person, because it seems that I've been thrust into a position of defending that view. I guess mine would be a two-stage response.

The first thing I would say is that it depends on how you define "the system". It seems that there are two aspects of this: the limits of your system and emergent properties. Suppose we think about a defective gene, and then you can isolate that because it's at the right level of the system that you're talking about. You could say, *"That's the faulty thing that is what's causing some molecular malfunction over here."* So we can look at some causal chain and point to that to try to remedy something: there's too much of this thing that releases a protein which has an inhibitory effect, or whatever.

To use your analogy of the computer with the virus, you can't just look at the ones and zeros changing in some weird way, because there's some higher-level process involved. That's analogous to all the different issues with reductionism. We all know that if you want to understand biological processes it doesn't really help to look at things from the order of quarks. There are some things that only happen at a sufficiently high level. So the virus would be an emergent property of sorts, and then you have all these problems regarding how that actually happens, but it clearly is a different thing on the systems level.

The virus that corrupts your computer is virtually impossible to explain in terms of the hardware of your computer, as you were saying. You have to somehow take an overarching systems view and say, *"This is an emergent thing which happened."* It's conceivable that we would know that the zeros and ones are corrupted, but the explanation for that would have to be at some emergent level.

The other point that I wanted to make from my category-one perspective with respect to something like PTSD is, *"Well, again that depends on how big your system is. Yes, absolutely the fact that you were shell shocked or experienced some stress event has to be incorporated within all the data that I have. That too is quantifiable. That too can be written in some reductionist code or as part of our system."*

VF: In terms of brain states?

HB: Yes. It seems to me that the impingement of the environment on our brain is part of the system and definitely has to be taken into account.

But of course there's a real difference between these philosophical discussions dealing with what's possible in principle and how you actually go about treating these things in practice: what one should actually be doing on the ground, as it were.

When we're talking about things like autism, ADHD, schizophrenia, or PTSD, I believe that, whatever our philosophical category-one or category-two orientations may be, it's not terribly relevant in the real world of actually trying to do something.

Maybe you think differently, but my belief is that in the real world of conducting experiments we have to be looking at the higher level and the lower level simultaneously. We have to be trying to do the best we can to see what's actually working. So from a pragmatic perspective, I'm not sure it should make any difference.

VF: I do agree with you. I think that's generally a safe approach to scientific investigation. You don't know how an understanding is eventually going to emerge.

One reason I feel it's important to try to get these ideas across is that I think there is a tendency to have a—I'm going to use a potentially strong term—to have a sort of "biological chauvinism" about this, to say that a physical or biological explanation of some psychological phenomenon has some scientific privilege or superiority to a "merely psychological" characterization.

I can understand where that comes from. I heard a great talk when I was a graduate student by the famous philosopher John Searle, where he wanted to argue that Cartesian dualism—an issue you brought up a little while ago—is alive and well and not just in certain quarters where we might not be so surprised to see it, but just sort of in everyday folk discourse.

The basic intuition that many of us have that a shopping addiction is different from, say, a heroin addiction, is perhaps a reflection of this Cartesian-style dualism. Many would say that a shopping addiction is "just a behaviour," so you should be able to control it, whereas heroin is different because "it's a physical substance that's responsible for this addiction".

I suspect that's where a lot of this comes from: this idea that the domain of thoughts, ideas, and behaviours, is malleable in a way that physical influences are not. If you take the point of view that the mind is a functional system that determines a physical organization—that the physical organization isn't the way it is to give rise to function, but rather it's the function that determines what the physical system is like—if you take that seriously, then you end up, I think, being able to do more of an all-hands-on-deck thing, where you can say, *Let's figure out both, at a functional level—how things seem to be operating and what's causing what to happen—at the same time that we look for biological correlates of these things to see if there's also a way of getting a foothold there.*

HB: That's a great point to end on. I'd like to thank you very much, Vic, for chatting with me. It's been a very enjoyable experience.

VF: Thank you. The feeling is mutual. That was a lot of fun and very, very interesting.

Questions for Discussion:

1. To what extent has this conversation influenced your thinking about language, the mind and the brain?

2. What do you think was the most interesting part of this wide-ranging conversation? The least interesting part?

The Limits of Consciousness

A conversation with Martin Monti

Introduction

The Collective Unconscious

Martin Monti spends a considerable amount of time around people who seem decidedly indifferent to his efforts.

It's not that Martin is an unsympathetic fellow, you understand, or a masochistic one—it's just that this engaging cognitive scientist has spent a good chunk of his burgeoning career carefully studying patients in a vegetative state: a severe consciousness disorder characterized by, as the Merck Manual puts it, "*an absence of responsiveness and awareness due to overwhelming dysfunction of the cerebral hemispheres.*"

The only difference, practically speaking, between being in a vegetative state and a coma, is that the former condition is accompanied by the appearance of wakefulness—that is, patients in the vegetative state sometimes have their eyes open for prolonged periods of time, as if awake. Typically, those in a vegetative state have first been in a coma. Sadly, most remain in that state for the rest of their lives.

Why would a dynamic, talented researcher such as Martin, spend so much of his time studying patients in such an intractably horrendous condition?

Well, one reason is that there seems to be considerably more to vegetative-state patients than first meets the eye. Up until recently, all behavioural tests had demonstrated that such patients seemed comprehensively unresponsive to any external stimuli—leading scientists to conclude that their cerebral cortex, the extensive outer layer of the brain largely response for higher brain functions, was completely inactive.

But most intriguingly, as Martin informed me, recent advances in brain-imaging technology tell a rather different story.

> *"It actually turns out that after 10 to 15 years of using neuroimaging to look directly into the brain and see what's happening, that a lot can be going on in the brain, a lot of activity in terms of cognitive faculties, even in the absence of consciousness."*

What sorts of things might be happening in the brains of such patients? Well, they might be reacting to light, colour, sounds, or smells. They might be able to distinguish between a well-formed versus scrambled version of an object. They might be able to distinguish between spatial representations and faces.

And while Martin is anxious to clarify that, *"None of this tells me that the patient is actually seeing or recognizing what that image is"*, all of our recently acquired neuroimaging data are certainly highly suggestive of a state of affairs that is a far cry from the complete absence of cortical activity that we thought we were facing.

That is certainly surprising. But then Martin and his colleagues probed deeper, using a technique known as "motor imaging". It turns out that just imagining performing certain actions leads to a measurable increase in activation of certain areas of the brain associated with those actions.

> *"I could ask you to imagine performing a motor behaviour: playing tennis is a perfect example. Just the act of imagining yourself playing tennis will activate parts of your brain that have to do with that motor behaviour.*

> *"If I ask you to imagine yourself playing tennis when I say the word 'tennis', and I notice that, once I say the word and your brain begins to activate in all these different areas that have to do with motor control, that tells me, as an outside observer, that you heard what I said, understood it, had enough memory available so that when you heard the word "tennis", you knew that meant that I'm asking you to imagine playing tennis and you were prepared to wilfully engage in that activity—that is, imagining yourself playing tennis."*

When Martin and his colleagues conducted similar tests with severely consciously-impaired patients, the results were little less than astounding, with similar, distinctly-recognizable brain-activation patterns occurring for a significant fraction of them.

> *"It actually turns out that in about 20% of patients who appear uncon-scious at the bedside—which is to say they can't show a wilful motoric response that is sufficient to persuade us of their consciousness—they **can** actually still do things with their brain."*

What does it all mean?

Well, for Martin, this is suggestive of the idea that our advanced technology has revealed that consciousness, which once appeared as a sharply-defined attribute that one either possessed or didn't, is in actuality vastly fuzzier.

> *"It's a spectrum. It's a very wide spectrum and we somewhat artifi-cially draw a line between who can show that they're conscious and who can't. That's where the line is today."*

Which brings us promptly to the larger question, *What is conscious-ness, really?* What is happening in our brains to allow it to occur in the first place? If it's not simply appropriate regions of cortical neurons firing when they should, what is it?

Martin doesn't have the answer yet, of course. But he believes that his research suggestively points towards reinforcing aspects of some recent concepts proposed by others, such as Giulio Tononi of the University of Wisconsin-Madison.

> *"Imagine your brain as a network of connected nodes that talk to each other and try to quantify how information flows in the brain. After all, the brain is really all about information exchange and processing between different areas, different neurons.*

> *"So we asked, 'If we take a perfectly healthy person who undergoes anaesthesia—that is, we artificially knock them out—how does*

information processing change in the brain? Do the properties of the network change?'

"There was something that we found that I thought was very striking. I found it profound, because it matches a theoretical proposal by Giulio Tononi: the data spontaneously almost exactly matched one of the many theories of consciousness we have.

"The main idea is that when you lose consciousness, the information exchange becomes extremely inefficient. One analogy that I've used in terms of the difference in neural function between being conscious and unconscious is that of driving directly from Los Angeles to New York as opposed to making the same trip in a bus, zigzagging between different towns and making all sorts of stops along the way.

"The one characteristic signature that we found of unconsciousness is that it is a very inefficient exchange of information.

"That led to thinking that consciousness might not be so much of a place, but more of a **mode***: a way in which information is exchanged; in particular, how information from different parts of the brain are brought together and integrated."*

Martin realizes all too well that we're still a long way from his quest to formulate a "mechanistic understanding" of consciousness. But after millennia of pondering and speculation, there are strong indications that we might, finally, be on the right track to a much deeper, more nuanced appreciation of what consciousness actually is.

And wouldn't it be fitting if a key piece to the riddle lay with those whom we were once convinced weren't actually conscious at all?

The Conversation

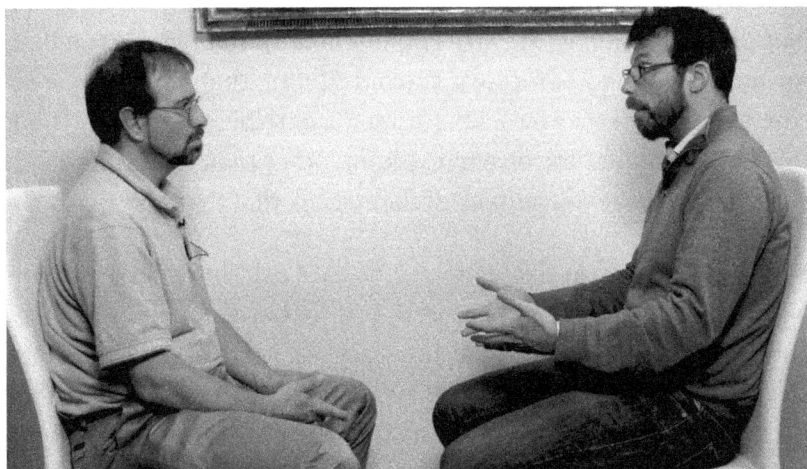

I. Dualism and Science Journalism

Changing hearts and brains

HB: I'm shortly going to be talking to a philosopher who believes strongly that the brain causes the mind, that the mind is simply a manifestation of brain states (see the Ideas Roadshow conversation *Philosophy of Brain* with Patricia Churchland). You were just telling me a moment ago before we started filming that you often start some of your courses by asking students whether or not they think that there's something else to the mind other than the brain, and a surprisingly large percentage of them think that there is.

MM: That's right. And keep in mind that I ask this question to an elite group of students. We're at UCLA, so these students are probably pretty educated and have done several years of studies before showing up in my class. But still, when I ask them if they think that there's something beyond the brain that causes who they are, I would say that typically about 80% of them say yes. That's, at the beginning of my class in dualism.

HB: Do you ask the question again at the end of your class?

MM: I do. And the answer does come down a little bit, usually to about 60/40. I can persuade about 20% of the students that that's not the case.

It's so ingrained in our culture that there is something beyond us, that there is something bigger. It feels so right, so natural.

Who controls my hands? Well, my brain. But the question is: Who does "*my*" refer to? Who is co-referential to "*my*"? I am my brain. The kind of arguments I typically give my students are somewhere along these lines. I show them, for example, that if something drastic changes in your brain, perhaps due to a brain injury, that will have very profound consequences on who you are.

HB: But surely everyone is aware of this at some level. They're aware of the changes that happen when they take psychotropic drugs, or even painkillers. We know that accidents to the brain can change personalities. What's going on, then, do you think? Is there some kind of compartmentalization for people? Some kind of denial?

MM: That is a difficult question, because if you think about it, this intuition has been deeply embedded in our culture until very recently.

Think about movies that you see. Neither you nor I have any real problems when a small kid supposedly goes to sleep and wakes up in the body of a grown actor. We have no problem imagining Lindsay Lohan's mind in somebody else's body. We even have no problem imagining that a spirit or demon could inhabit my body and take over who I am. This is so just embedded everywhere in our culture. It's embedded in our language when we say "*my hand*", as opposed to "*my brain*". The difference is that you can change anything about your body except your brain, and still be you.

I could undergo plastic surgery and get a better nose or stronger cheekbones, but it would still be me. The one thing that can't change without affecting who "*me*" is, is my brain.

HB: Right. We cling on to this tenaciously. Let me move to a slightly different subject. There are certainly many reasons to believe that neuroscience is becoming increasingly popular these days. There are an awful lot of articles and popularizations of cognitive science around, together with speculations on what the future might hold.

You yourself have participated in some of these popularizations: you've written articles and given talks, and you engage quite regularly with the public. Do you think that, as a general rule, people are getting the right message? Do they understand what is happening on the cutting edge of neuroscience and psychology these days, or are they missing things, are they confused?

MM: Well, I get the feeling that people mostly get a sort of dreamy version of what is happening, the sexy wording of what's happening, which often leaves out the details that are so crucial to what the real finding is.

For example, one newspaper headline that came out of a study that I published some years ago was, *Scientist speaks with dead person*. Of course, we did not talk with anybody who is dead—nothing could be further away from the truth. But it was probably more appealing to the headline writer, in the hopes of grabbing the attention of the readership.

Now, I myself spend a lot of time trying to explain to journalists what I think is happening. Who else should be doing that, if not myself? It's *my* study, after all, and I'm probably the one who knows the most details about it and how best to interpret it. So I do spend a fair amount of time trying to explain or correct some common misconceptions, so that journalists—who are, by definition, not specialists in my discipline—can try to disseminate the clearest and most accurate message possible.

After all, just imagine it from their perspective, facing an editor who demands, "*By tomorrow morning I need a 500-word article on the vegetative state*," and perhaps they have no real experience whatsoever with the topic.

HB: So if I'm a member of the general public and I want to know what's new in cognitive science or psychology, where would you recommend that I go?

MM: I would look into actual press releases from the university and the scientists themselves. Many specialist journals would be very good as well. Both *Science* and *Nature*, for example, have their own podcasts. You could have a podcast on your phone and just listen to the 5 or 10 most interesting studies in whatever you're interested in. I would probably recommend getting my information from there, rather than the regular press.

Questions for Discussion:

1. Do you believe that the mind is more than "just" the brain?

2. Do you think that, over time, the mainstream media will simply refer people to popular reviews of current research produced by the likes of **Science** *or* **Nature** *rather than trying to do science journalism themselves? Should they?*

II. Inside The Other

A constant concern

HB: I'd like to eventually turn to the vegetative state and your research there, but first I'd like to back up and ask you more generally how you got into the field to begin with.

My understanding is that you've had a bit of a double tack to get here. You started off in classical languages and literature, then you went into economics, and you eventually ended up in cognitive science. Is there any field of study that you haven't considered seriously?

MM: Well, I certainly have very varied interests. Retrospectively, I can say that there is a certain coherence to the path itself.

HB: So what is that, exactly?

MM: I vividly remember wondering, between middle school and high school, whether what I was seeing was exactly the same as what other people were seeing. It might seem very simplistic, but of course I was a child at that point.

HB: Maybe you were a solipsist.

MM: It's possible.

I was wondering if whatever colour I was seeing, for example, felt the same way to someone else. So I might see orange one way, and you might see it in a completely different way, but we just both agree that is orange and call it that way.

HB: By convention.

MM: Right, exactly: by convention. I was trying, in a sense, to wrap my head around what might have been convention versus what might have been reality, and the interplay between the two.

In high school, I was first exposed to these issues in philosophy, and I was naturally attracted to that and found it particularly interesting—not only philosophy of mind, but also the classical philosophers, who were so often wondering what is real and what is not.

How can we ever know what is real or not? All I have to rely on around me are my own senses. In a sense, I never have the benefit of being outside of my brain to appreciate what the world really looks like.

I found these arguments particularly interesting and worthy of study. Somewhat more concretely, this led me to study how people make choices and how we make decisions when we don't know what is likely to happen: choice under uncertainty.

What I found particularly interesting was how we had the presumption to fit people's decisions into mathematical equations. I spent a lot of time writing and thinking about dynamical systems that would somehow explain how equilibria shifted in markets, how people would make decisions.

HB: This sounds to me like classical economic thinking: maximizing utility functions and all that kind of stuff.

MM: Exactly. This starts from the second half of the 19th century, with people like Léon Walras talking about "expected utility": we choose our actions based on what gives us the highest probable pleasure.

HB: That's all wrong, you know.

MM: That was also my intuition. I thought, *"But people **don't** really do this."* And that's what led me to study the mind: I wanted to know how people *actually* make decisions, which led me to a PhD in psychology and neuroscience.

And while I was doing that, I started developing my interest for what are probably two of the more characterizing aspects of the human mind: language and consciousness. They may not be unique to us, but they are certainly the most characterizing features of our cognitive system.

HB: I must say, there actually *is* an extremely coherent thread throughout your personal history, the way you presented it. Perhaps you've been working on the story.

MM: Well, hindsight is 20-20.

HB: So, tell me how you got involved with research in the vegetative state in particular. I'd like to talk more generally about consciousness, but first I'd like to specifically discuss your work with the vegetative state and minimally conscious states. Tell me how you got particularly involved in that, and then we can back up and start defining terms a little bit.

MM: Sure. While pursuing my doctoral studies I had the opportunity to look into other aspects of what was called "cognitive neuroscience". It was partly due to some requirements I had during my doctoral studies that allowed me to look beyond what I was doing at the time—which I still do, in parallel, with my current research.

HB: So this was your work on language?

MM: That's right. I started with language in my doctoral studies. The very first paper I wrote was in experimental decision-making, experimental economics; and from there we moved into how people reason. And then I began to wonder whether or not language plays some sort of a deep role in our very complicated reasoning process.

In parallel with this, I was required to explore other aspects of the field that I might find interesting. That is what led me to discover a very small field, which at the time was only being studied by two or three people at most. It concerned patients who lose consciousness, all the while without even having a definition of what consciousness is in the scientific sense of a definition. I found that extremely interesting.

How do you know if someone is conscious? I wish I had a thermometer that I could put in somebody's ear and say, "*Oh, 100: they're conscious.*" But we don't.

The deep question is that sometimes you're forced to decide whether or not someone else is conscious. How do we do that? If you're judging your own consciousness, it's very easy: you have access to the feeling—whatever the feeling turns out to be in reality—which is what you have learned to call consciousness.

It's this kind of self-reflection or sense of agency: a sense of experiencing the world. So it's easy for you to say about yourself, "*I'm conscious.*" It's easy for me to say it about myself. But it's really hard for you to say that *I* am conscious. You can't say it for sure—you can never be certain, because you don't have access to my feelings of agency, experience, and so forth.

That's what got me particularly interested in this field: *How can we ever get to know if someone else is conscious?*

HB: This seems to me to be strikingly reminiscent of your question as a small child, of whether something is really orange—you can't get inside someone's head, as it were.

MM: That's right. I'm coming full circle.

Questions for Discussion:

1. Why do you think that Howard and Martin are sceptical of the classical economic notion of rational decision-making?

2. Do you think that we will ever reach a stage where we will develop a "thermometer for consciousness" and be able to objectively determine another person's consciousness? What might that look like?

III. The Vegetative State
Evolving understanding

HB: Before we talk about the vegetative state and how it relates to aspects of consciousness, let's first talk about what a vegetative state *is*. I'm guessing that many non-specialists will make an automatic equivalence between a vegetative state and a coma, but that's actually not correct.

MM: Yes. A vegetative state is a neurological condition in which at least one of the two cardinal elements of consciousness is affected. For example, a vegetative patient is someone who appears awake, at least inasmuch as his eyes open and close in cycles. Such patients give the impression of waking up and falling asleep just as much as you or I do. Whether they truly wake up or fall asleep is a different question.

So they do *seem* awake, but they don't show any sign of being conscious of themselves or what's happening around them. That is a vegetative state. Essentially it's wakefulness in the absence of awareness.

A coma is a circumstance where a patient doesn't have any awareness of himself and also does not appear to be awake. In a sense, you can think of a coma as a step below a vegetative state. Normally the way in which you would enter this condition is by a very severe brain injury, by an accident or an aneurysm or something like that. A patient may get into a coma, which typically means that the eyes are closed, and the patient doesn't show any sign of being aware.

This is very similar to what happens in general anaesthesia: you're completely out. People don't like calling anaesthesia coma, but that's essentially what it is from a brain point of view.

Some awake from a coma without recovering consciousness—wakefulness without awareness—and that is a vegetative state. Now some of these patients also move on to recover some level of awareness, and that's when they enter a minimally conscious state.

It's very easy for me to tell if a patient is in a coma or a vegetative state, because in a comatose patient the eyes are always closed, whereas in a vegetative state the eyes are either open or closed, depending on the wakefulness of the patient.

What is really difficult is how to determine whether or not a patient who is awake has regained that little bit of consciousness sufficient for me to say, *"Now, the patient is at least minimally conscious."*

That's where the real debate is. And that's also the debate that society is having, generally, about these sorts of patients.

HB: But even before we get into full-blown consciousness, one of the intriguing things that you've done is to more subtly parse what we mean by consciousness, by examining what is going on in the brains of those in a vegetative state, examining what such patients might be feeling or seeing, or, more generally to what extent they are experiencing brain activity.

It seems to me that some time ago there was a general belief throughout the neuroscientific community that virtually nothing was happening within the brains of patients in a vegetative state.

MM: Absolutely. In fact, particularly in Europe, the vegetative state has often been used synonymously with the apallic syndrome—the word, "apallic", from Latin, meaning, "without a pallium", with the pallium being the cortex. These patients, then, were literally believed not to be experiencing any cortical activity. That's why we call it the vegetative state: the functions that allow the body to remain alive are sufficiently preserved.

For example, these patients are not typically on a ventilator. So when people think about pulling the plug on a patient, there isn't actually a plug to pull here. They're alive and they remain alive, they just don't seem to express that feeling of consciousness.

As I said, there was a long-standing belief that these patients don't seem to have a functioning cortex. It actually turns out, after 10 to 15 years of using neuroimaging to look directly into the brain and see what's happening, that a lot can be going on in the brain, a lot of activity in terms of cognitive faculties, even in the absence of consciousness.

For example, for someone who is either sleeping or in a vegetative state, her brain may still react to a sound heard from the outside. The brain might respond appropriately to sounds from the environment, but that doesn't necessarily mean that those who are sleeping, or in a vegetative state, are actually hearing.

HB: But *something* is going on. I understand that you can't just assume that all the processes are the same as someone who is awake and hearing, but you can see that there is *some* activity; and previously the common belief was that there was nothing.

MM: Absolutely. And this is what I believe is the very first revolution in this field: finding out that these brains that we thought were not functioning at the level of the cortex, actually are. The question is, *How much?*

Questions for Discussion:

1. To what extent can we distinguish from the brain responding to stimuli from "outside" or "inside"?

2. Why do you think, exactly, that "people don't like calling anaesthesia coma"? Might this be related to the widespread belief, mentioned earlier, in the distinction between the mind and the brain? To what extent do you think that deliberately opting to refer to anaesthesia as "sleep" is associated with this issue?

IV. Probing Vegetative States

Some experimental details

HB: What, exactly, are you testing, and how do you do it? You mentioned auditory stimuli, but I understand that you're also looking at visual and tactile stimuli, and you even have tests for language.

MM: These days we're using a number of different tools to try to look at brain processing in these patients. The most widely employed would be electroencephalography (EEG), which is normally a cap that somebody can wear in which there are electrodes that can capture the presence of small magnetic fields created by a number of neurons all working together at the same time.

What I use most often is functional magnetic resonance imaging (fMRI). This is a technique where, rather than directly capturing some aspect of neuronal function, one looks at the energetic fingerprint of those functions. If we use a certain part of the brain for some process, more blood is sent towards that part of the brain to replenish nutrients and essentially bring energy.

Those are the two most common ways of tracking brain activity.

Now, the basic level of these sorts of experiments would be to play sounds, say, and analyze how differently the brain responds to a sound versus silence. What we can determine from a study like this is whether or not the neuronal circuitry is functioning.

Getting slightly more sophisticated, I can play sentences that are in English versus sounds that are not. Then if I find a difference in activation in specific parts of the brain, which suggests that this brain is recognizing the difference between language as an organized type of utterance versus just any sound.

You can imagine making this more and more complicated. One study we did on vision was essentially a staircase, starting from the very simple question of whether or not the brains of these patients respond to light, then moving on to considering motion or colour. Do the brains of these patients recognize that certain categories of stimuli are different?

For example, you can show a well-formed object versus a scrambled version of that object. Some parts of our brains are particularly interested in coherent objects—like a telephone or an alarm clock—and you can notice whether or not this part of the brain gets engaged when they are presented with coherent versions of objects versus a scrambled version of those same things.

Then you can keep moving on up to, say, pictures of faces versus pictures of houses. There are parts of our brains that are particularly interested in spatial locations, and others that are particularly interested in faces. I can show a picture of a face to a patient and see if the corresponding part of the brain becomes metabolically active, for example. And that tells me that the brain is working.

However, I should stress that none of this tells me if the patient is actually seeing or recognizing what that image is.

HB: Do you ever get any feedback afterwards from these people? I can imagine there are some people who are in a vegetative state while you're doing these experiments, they're in a fMRI machine or what have you, and then they regain consciousness and perhaps can then remember the tests that you performed.

MM: No. These are the cases that are most advertised in the media, but they are not what typically happens. On top of that there's an interesting question: if somebody tells you that they have a recollection, is that a real recollection or is it a dream, a distortion of what actually happened?

HB: Sure. But perhaps you could filter that out with statistics.

MM: I don't think we would have sufficient numbers.

HB: How often does this actually happen, that people become conscious after having been in a vegetative state?

MM: Well, I've been working in this field for several years now and it still hasn't happened to me.

HB: Not often, then.

MM: In fairness, I typically see patients only once or twice: perhaps the families move away or something.

I think that where the science is today is in trying to take one snapshot of these patients and try to understand what is happening. There are other questions, such as those you raised, like, *How much that happens during this stage can then influence behaviour at a later point if they regain consciousness?* But I just don't think we've gotten there yet.

Questions for Discussion:

1. Why do you think that Martin makes such an emphatic distinction between recognizing common brain activation areas and a conclusion that the patient is actually seeing or recognizing something?

2. How likely do you think it will be that, as neuroscience progresses, greater percentages of those with severe brain injuries will begin to recover consciousness (broadly defined)?

V. Beyond Reflex

A thin line

HB: What are the practical, ethical aspects of this, in terms of getting permission to participate in these sorts of experiments? Do people sign something like an organ donor card in advance, should they find themselves in a horrible car accident? Or does it happen in some other way?

For the record, I should say that I'm all in favour of you doing stuff on me, by the way, should I somehow be in that situation, because I'd really like you guys to fix me, which will likely only happen if people like you continue to do your experiments and find out what's going on. But I'm just curious to know how all that works.

MM: Sure. As a scientist, I'm bound to some kind of institution that oversees and approves anything I do, like an Institutional Review Board or Institutional Review Panel. Each university has its own panel, which is normally comprised of some scientists and members of the public. In practice, this means that anything I do with these patients is evaluated before I ever do it. The main aim of that is to avoid circumstances where I do something that may have either negative repercussions or where there's any potential risk. My studies need to show, typically, that there is something to be learned in the absence of any significant risk to the patient.

Now the question that you are raising is who is allowed to say yes to a patient's participation, when the patients are obviously unable to agree themselves. Normally there is somebody legally responsible, a next of kin or someone placed by a judge to be the representative. I cannot perform any experiment unless I collect the written assent of the patient's legal representative.

HB: Are these people typically in a situation where they've been in a vegetative state for a long period of time?

MM: You can look at patients during different moments of their condition. For example, most of what I've done so far was with chronic patients, those who have been in a vegetative state from anywhere from a few months to several years. Many studies look at these chronic populations.

Currently, however, I'm interested in acute patients, which means that I'm mostly looking at comatose patients or very early vegetative-state patients. The reason for that is because now that I know that even in chronic patients so much can be going on in their brains, I'd like to be able to take a snapshot of somebody the first day after some kind of brain injury and be able to tell what are their chances of recovery, what can we do to help them recover and so forth.

Most of the literature you will find on this is in chronic patients though.

HB: So I'm guessing that, from your perspective, the idea is that if you can build up sufficient amounts of data from those who have just entered a vegetative state, you can then later match up their brain imaging records with their health trajectory to better determine what is going on, what their chances for recovery might be, and so forth.

MM: Absolutely. In fact, the mission of my lab today is to develop some kind of mechanistic understanding of the physiology of consciousness. *Why do we have consciousness in the first place? How, exactly, do we sometimes lose it? Why and how do some people recover it?*

My dream for the endpoint of this segment of my research would be exactly that: I would love to have a physiological model of how the brain supports consciousness and what parts of this model break down following a brain injury. In principle, then, I could take a picture from the very first day following an accident so as to tell what part of the circuitry is broken—metaphorically speaking—and how we might somehow intervene to further the chances of the patient actually recovering.

HB: Technically, what is the difference between a vegetative state and a minimally conscious state? I'm guessing minimally conscious means that we're moving up towards consciousness, but how would you define it?

MM: Well, using standard clinical tools you would be at the bedside of these patients, and you would try to get them to reveal to you that they're conscious. Now, I wish that I could just somehow look into their brain and feel their sense of consciousness, but I can't. So what we typically do is try to get them to produce any kind of behaviour that would convince us that they are conscious.

For example, during this conversation, you've probably inferred that it's very likely that I'm conscious. You might think that we are in some kind of *Matrix* where nothing is really as it seems, but I would guess that you are mostly persuaded that I am conscious.

HB: More than "mostly", I'd say.

MM: The question, though, is *why*? ***What***, specifically, is convincing you that I'm conscious? Probably it's because I'm behaving in ways that are not entirely reflexive: I produce behaviour that somehow reveals the presence of an agent, some conscious agent.

And that's exactly what we do in the clinic: we go to the bedside and we ask the patient to maybe move a hand, or to blink his or her eyes, and we try to elicit any possible form of wilful behaviour.

The problem is that often people move in reflexive ways, just like when the doctor taps your patella and your leg extends. There's no consciousness there, it's just a circuit. Now how do you distinguish between the conscious motion and the reflexive motion? That's the big problem.

It actually turns out to be pretty difficult: people can make very complicated motions that are purely the result of patterns stored in their brain. You might often see patients do very complicated things, but they're entirely reflexive.

I'll never forget one case I had which was very early on in my career, the patient was sitting in his chair and was very clearly sleeping, while my colleague and I were preparing to do one of these tests.

The patient's eyes suddenly opened, he stretched his arms, yawned, and then shifted over to the other side of the chair. But other than that, we couldn't get this patient to show *any* sign of consciousness when we asked him to move his hand, blink, look towards us or whatever. We could get *no* sign of wilful consciousness from this person.

So here we are, left to wonder, *If a patient can wake up, yawn, stretch, find a more comfortable position in his chair, is that a sign of consciousness?* It's tough.

That's what's so complicated: so much of our behaviour is purely reflexive, which in many ways is great. Imagine if you had to consciously focus on any single behaviour that you did. Think about how often you drive without fully focusing on it, preoccupied with other thoughts, steering and changing gears automatically. Imagine if you had to fully focus on all those tasks all the time. It would be overwhelming.

Imagine if, right now as you're looking at me, you had to consciously process the lines that make up my face and say, "*Oh, that's a face.*" It just happens for you. There's so much of that which is happening in your brain that it's tough to tell what is conscious and what is not.

Questions for Discussion:

1. What, exactly, do you think Martin means by a "mechanistic model for the physiology of consciousness"? What sorts of things would be necessary to learn in order to build such a model?

2. What do you think is the evolutionary justification for the large amount of "reflex activity" that we exhibit?

3. To what extent would a complete "mechanistic model of the physiology of consciousness" as per #1 above necessarily account for how some of our oft-repeated behaviour becomes "reflexive"?

VI. Assessing Consciousness

Unlikely tennis players

HB: I'd like to return for a moment to the fact that people used to believe that the brain was dormant, that when you're in a vegetative state, basically nothing was going on in the cerebral cortex and just the basic bodily functions were being supported.

My sense is that the breakthrough that researchers like yourself have discovered is that there are varying levels of activity for different sorts of stimuli, so much so that it seems that what previously seemed like an on/off switch for consciousness is now regarded as a continuum, a spectrum; and that over the last 15–20 years science has been steadily filling in this gap so that we can't draw the line nearly as sharply as we used to. Is that a fair assessment?

MM: Absolutely. You've used the right word: it's a spectrum. It's a very wide spectrum, and we somewhat artificially draw a line between who can show that they're conscious and who can't. That's where the line is today.

Now, embedded in these words is a very clear problem. What if someone were conscious, but just could not say, *"I'm here."* Maybe she has some kind of motor impairment that prevents her from moving her hands when asked. And that's where what I typically think of as the second revolution of brain imaging comes into play.

Maybe you can't produce behaviour that would convince me that you're conscious, so you can't overtly move or respond to commands, but maybe I can ask you to wilfully do something with your brain.

That is, it's not just the case of me looking at your brain when I'm playing sounds and see if it responds, but instead I would ask you to do a specific mental task, and then I would actually see the fingerprint of that in your brain. Then that would be sufficient enough for me to infer that there is agency in you, which is where we draw the line.

HB: And you have been doing these kinds of experiments. You've conducted experiments where you've had people imagine playing tennis.

MM: Right. The motivation behind these experiments is exactly this: imagine a patient was lying there, perfectly conscious but unable to move. How would we ever know, just looking from the outside, that this patient is actually conscious? It would be impossible. You could never infer that there was an agent.

But maybe, although he can't do anything motor-related, he can do something with his mind. The intuition that led to this is something very simple. I could ask you to imagine performing a motor behaviour: playing tennis is a perfect example. Just the act of imagining yourself playing tennis will activate parts of your brain that have to do with that motor behaviour.

If I ask you to imagine yourself playing tennis when I say the word "tennis", and I notice that, once I say the word and your brain begins to activate in all these different areas that have to do with motor control, that tells me, as an outside observer, that you heard what I said, understood it, had enough memory available so that when you heard the word "tennis", you knew that meant that I'm asking you to imagine playing tennis, and you were prepared to wilfully engage in that activity—that is, imagining yourself playing tennis.

HB: And you've done precisely these sorts of experiments on some of your patients.

MM: Yes, we've done these sorts of experiments; and it actually turns out that in about 20% of patients who appear unconscious at the bedside—which is to say they can't show a wilful motoric response that is sufficient to persuade us of their consciousness— they can *still* do things with their brain.

So this leaves us in a slightly uncertain position, where the tests that we thought were so good at understanding if someone is conscious or not, are still very good, but now there's also this grey area.

HB: By tests, you mean, the previous behavioural tests?

MM: That's right, exactly.

HB: And now you've been able to push the boundaries considerably using these new brain-imaging tests.

MM: Yes.

HB: When I hear you describe this, it strikes me as very much analogous to this fictional thermometer that you were talking about earlier.

Assuming that the technology is good enough to get a clear signal of what is going on, if these people hear the word "tennis" and then there's a subsequent display of neural activity in their motor regions equivalent to that of an unimpaired person when subjected to the same conditions, I'm personally ready to conclude that this patient is conscious. I don't have the slightest doubt whatsoever about that.

Which tells me that there's a misdiagnosis, I guess you could say, or an incomplete diagnosis compared to what was done just using the previous behavioural conditions, for those 20% of people. However you want to call it, exactly, that seems to me a huge enhancement in our understanding of what's actually going on.

MM: Yes. It's not a misdiagnosis in the technical sense, because the doctor who made the previous diagnosis did everything right. It's more a limit of the way we're using behaviour as a proxy for consciousness. You can have consciousness and not have behaviour, and you'd miss that without these enhanced techniques.

In a sense, this technique allows us to infer even better. Those grey areas are a little bit clearer than before. However, you could imagine that our tests would fail if you were perfectly conscious but couldn't move and couldn't understand language.

HB: In other words, it's a sufficient demonstration of consciousness but it's not a necessary proof of consciousness.

MM: Exactly. If someone can engage in imaginary tennis when we ask him to, that must mean he's conscious. But if you can't, it's just a negative result. It could be that he didn't hear us, he didn't want to do it, or was sleeping—

HB: Or doesn't play tennis?

MM: I should say—I've been asked this many times—that even if you don't know how to play tennis you still get that corresponding activation in your motor areas.

Questions for Discussion:

1. *The notion of a "spectrum" in cognitive science is gaining favour in a number of different areas of cognitive science, from autism to schizophrenia to consciousness. Do you think this represents a growing understanding of the nature of the brain, an awareness of the limitations of previous definitions or a form of fashion?*

2. *Are you as convinced as Martin and Howard seem to be that a patient who consistently activates motor neurons associated with tennis when asked to imagine playing tennis is conscious? Might this, too, be a specific type of "reflex" that was mentioned earlier?*

VII. Extracting Information
Two types of controls

HB: I'd like to discuss some details about how these neuroimaging studies are actually done. We were talking before about fMRI as a technique to measure blood flow to certain regions of the brain, where increased blood flow in a particular region corresponds to increased neural activity, but of course we know that the brain is normally active all the time, so in order to do these experiments properly we need some baseline of ambient neural activity from which we can subtract.

MM: Absolutely.

HB: That I already knew. But what I hadn't really thought about until I read some of your work is the tremendous amount of attention that is often required towards finding the right sort of questions and techniques to experimentally assess that baseline and measure changes in specific regions.

MM: Yes. The problem is actually analogous to the problem I was mentioning before of recognizing what part of motor behaviour is conscious and what part is reflexive.

Your brain, as you correctly said, is active all the time. Even when you're sleeping, your brain is active. Most of your brain's activities are beyond your control: you have no say into whether this or that part of your brain is active.

So the way we've been using these techniques for studies is twofold.

One I was mentioning earlier: if I played two different sounds to you—just noise and language, say—I can subtract the basic activity of your brain of just hearing noise from the activity that it takes your brain to recognize language. If there is any difference between these two activities, this tells me that your brain has done something slightly different—which, in turn tells me that your brain is recognizing language as such. This is one way of doing it.

The other way of doing it, which is the way we do it with the tennis example, has a different philosophy. In that case I give you exactly the same stimulation, but I ask you to do different things with it. Your brain is receiving the same amount of environmental stimulation, but you're doing different things with it.

There's one experiment that we recently published that went something like this. You're in the fMRI machine and all that you're hearing is one word every second, so you're hearing sequences of twenty-six words, and some of these words repeat.

Either I don't say anything to you and you just listen to the words, or I explicitly ask you to count the number of times a given word repeats.

That is, the stimulation—the strings of words—is identical, what's coming in is identical, but if you are indeed conscious and you're complying with my instructions, the mental activity that is ongoing is completely different: you're remembering, you're monitoring, you're counting, and so forth.

So if I see a physical difference between a condition in which the stimulation is identical but the mindset is different, then I have a fingerprint of you wilfully doing something.

Questions for Discussion:

1. How can we be certain that the two techniques Martin mentions in this chapter are equally effective in all cases? Might some techniques be more effective with particular individuals or particular cases?

2. To what extent do you think these techniques would have significantly diminished effectiveness for those who had difficulty focusing or following instructions? What, if anything, do you think this would imply regarding particular challenges associated with using neuroimaging techniques to study conditions like ADHD?

VIII. Quantifying Consciousness

Towards more rigorous models

HB: Let's move on to a broader discussion of consciousness in general. You're examining patients in a range of severe brain-injury cases as a probe in order to get a clear sense of where the threshold of consciousness is.

But my understanding is that you also have some ideas of how we might explicitly clarify and categorize the connections within the brain by using some aspects of mathematics, such as graph theory. This seems like a really intriguing idea to me, and one that might help bring us closer to some form of a testable hypothesis to probe consciousness.

After all, consciousness is one of those thorny issues that philosophers have been talking about for millennia, but perhaps science is starting to develop empirical and theoretical procedures whereby we can finally begin moving more concretely towards a deeper understanding of things.

MM: Of course the ultimate goal is to have a scientific definition of what consciousness is. Today in my view the best definition comes from an Italian scientist, Giulio Tononi, who says that consciousness is the thing that goes away when you go into dreamless sleep and comes back when you wake in the morning. That is pretty much as good a definition as we have in scientific terms.

We don't yet have a tangible, objective way of defining it, which we would obviously love to have. So a big effort that is happening today—and the studies you mentioned are precisely part of that effort—is to ask if we can somehow *quantify* consciousness. Can we assign *numbers* to brain processes? Can we somehow find this thermometer that I've been talking about, this way of quantifying what's happening?

One way of doing it is to imagine your brain as a network of connected nodes that talk to each other and try to quantify how information flows in the brain. After all, the brain is really all about information exchange and processing between different areas, different neurons.

So we asked ourselves, If we take a perfectly healthy person who undergoes anaesthesia—that is, we artificially knock them out—how does information processing change in the brain? Do the properties of the network change?

There was something that we found that I thought was very striking. I found it profound, because it matches a theoretical proposal by Giulio Tononi: the data spontaneously almost exactly matched one of the many theories of consciousness we have.

The main idea is that when you lose consciousness, the information exchange becomes extremely inefficient. One analogy that I've used in terms of the difference in neural function between being conscious and unconscious is that of driving directly from Los Angeles to New York as opposed to making the same trip in a bus, zigzagging between different towns and making all sorts of stops along the way.

The one characteristic signature that we found of unconsciousness is that it is a very inefficient exchange of information.

That led to thinking that consciousness might not be so much of a place, but more of a *mode*: a way in which information is exchanged—in particular, how information from different parts of the brain are brought together and integrated.

HB: When you say inefficient, what do you mean by that? You mean something analogous to this zigzagging, but what, more specifically, do you mean?

MM: Imagine I had a note in my pocket that I wanted to give to you. I could simply hand it to you from here and that would be extremely efficient. Alternatively I could give this note to someone else and they could go to a friend of yours, give it to them, and eventually it would arrive to you, which is a much more inefficient way of communication.

HB: So we're talking about distance measures, it seems: I have a region of the brain here that wants to talk to a region of the brain over there, and it's not taking the shortest path.

MM: Exactly. It's not taking the shortest path. It's forced to go other ways through different areas of the brain in order to reach its ultimate goal.

HB: So the hypothesis is that it's forced to go out of its way because the more directly-connected regions aren't sufficiently active?

MM: That's a very good question. The working hypothesis is that what's happening is that there's a certain circuit in the brain that allows long-range communication to happen very efficiently. This is a circuit that goes from particular areas of our cortex through the thalami—two nut-shaped regions in the very middle of your brain—back to other areas of the cortex, which allows for very efficient information exchange between two areas of the cortex that are far away from each other. It's kind of like a shortcut.

HB: So this capitalizes on the three-dimensional aspect of the brain, as it were.

MM: Yes. But not only that: also the fact that there is a direct connection between the cortex and the thalamus, and then from the thalamus back to other areas in the cortex.

HB: So it's not only where these regions are geographically located, but also how strong the throughput is from place to place?

MM: Exactly. One current theory is that there is a specific part of these thalami that receives and reciprocates connections to both the frontal and posterior part of your brain. And this circuit from the back of your brain, through the thalamus, to the front of your brain and back again is what allows information from very distant parts of your brain to be pulled together at the same time. 'Integration' is the word that people typically use.

Today there is a group of scientists who think of consciousness as "integrated information": being able to bring together information from very distant parts of your brain and put it together to create more information than you started with. According to some people, that is what consciousness is.

HB: So my sense is that there's a continuum of those who have lots of activity going on in their cortex—normal people—down to those who have a vastly diminished amount of activity—say, those in a vegetative state.

And at some point, if there's enough activity, connections are made between distant regions; and some emergent structure, or threshold is reached that we call "consciousness". Is that what we're saying here?

MM: I would rephrase that very slightly. Instead of focusing on the amount of activity in the cortex, I would put more emphasis on the connection between different areas. It is conceivable to have a perfectly preserved cortex that doesn't have these long-range connections and you would thus be unconscious.

There's one famous case, published in 1999, that has particularly puzzled most of the scientists in the domain of vegetative state and disorders of consciousness.

It concerns a lady who was in a very chronic vegetative state—in my recollection, it was between 5 and 10 years—but every now and then she said individual words.

My thinking is that what was probably happening was that the part of cortex that has to do with language was still active in an insular way, so it could still produce behaviour. But because there wasn't this integration of information, consciousness never arose. A functioning cortex is not sufficient to allow consciousness to arise: you need to have this integration.

HB: So I can imagine that by combining these various key features you're talking about—specific brain regions, strength of connections, associated neural circuitry you can begin modelling things by using some mathematical structure, weighting or network/circuitry mapping.

There should be a possibility in the future to flesh out a more comprehensive description of this architecture using various mathematical techniques.

MM: Exactly. What we've been doing right now is attempting a mathematical description of how a brain network changes as one goes in and out of consciousness. Of course, now we're trying to apply this to patients to see whether we can distinguish systematically patients who have had very similar brain injuries, but some might be conscious and some might not.

The term that I've been using most with the researchers and students in my lab is a quest to develop a "mechanistic understanding" of what's happening. We have correlations, we can see the numbers change in different states, but what I really want is to be able to draw boxes and arrows, give numbers and weights to explain communication across the brain, so that I can understand precisely that if I cut the circuit here or there, then I'm necessarily going to induce unconsciousness.

And then, of course, if you flip that way of thinking around, it means that if I can fully appreciate where a circuit is compromised, I can try to intervene and fix it. If only we could get this kind of mechanistic understanding of the physiological fingerprint of consciousness, then I could come up with ways for reigniting it.

Maybe it wouldn't always work. I can imagine cases where the system is so compromised that there is nothing we can do. For example, if the physical pathways were too compromised, there might be nothing I could reignite. But if the physical connections are not too compromised, maybe there's some way of facilitating the return of function.

HB: Relatedly, it seems to me that the more accurate models are developed, presumably, the better our diagnostic ability to determine whether or not people actually have much more consciousness than we've given them credit for up to now. In time, we could imagine probing them not only using the techniques you've mentioned—imagining playing tennis and so forth—but by directly examining the underlying mathematical network architecture that you and others are developing.

Once we have a more coherent measure of consciousness, we might even imagine additional ways to assist them in communicating with us, such as by using brain-machine interfaces.

MM: Absolutely. Certainly we're getting better and better at estimating how much brain function is left. I don't imagine that we'll one day find out that all patients who are in a vegetative state are, in fact, conscious. I feel quite confident in saying that those who are represent only a small minority. And the more we can develop these techniques, the better we will be at distinguishing between patients who have consciousness and those who do not.

In terms of what you were just saying, that's one of the steps that's actually being taken right now. I was involved in a large European grant that was investigating how we could use brain computer interfaces for patients to at least regain a small amount of their ability to interact with the environment.

Now we know that some patients can imagine playing tennis, for example, and this also applies to patients who we know are conscious but have completely limited mobility. These minimally-conscious patients shouldn't be thought of like us: they fluctuate in and out of consciousness.

But maybe by interacting with a machine, we can devise ways of having these people sometimes interact with us: turn on the TV, call someone, tell us they're hungry, and so forth. People are working very intensely on that. There's still an awful lot to do, but some results are now coming out.

Questions for Discussion:

1. How can we be certain that we are using the right approach to evaluate what we mean by "information" in the brain?

2. How might we use brain-machine interfaces to rigorously test specific models of consciousness? Those interested in more details of brain-machine interfaces are referred to **Minds and Machines**, *the Ideas Roadshow conversation with neuroscientist Miguel Nicolelis.*

IX. Interdisciplinary Interlude

Mathematics, cognitive science and other issues

HB: As you move towards developing a deeper understanding of the mathematical structure of this network architecture are there increasing opportunities to collaborate directly with mathematicians? Are there increasing opportunities for interdisciplinary activity? Or is it the case right now that many of these models have already been developed and it's more a question of assessing what already exists than developing new structures.

MM: Science has become so interdisciplinary in the last twenty years, particularly cognitive neuroscience. I couldn't do anything I'm doing today without the input from computer scientists, mathematicians and statisticians.

As we've been saying, graph theory, which is a branch of mathematics that has no reason to be connected to psychology and neuroscience, turns out, in fact, to be an extremely helpful way of thinking about the brain.

Particularly when it comes to these complicated questions, but I would even say across the board in the field of brain studies, the science is becoming increasingly interdisciplinary.

HB: One further question before we leave this topic. I hear about doctors deliberately putting people into comas as a medical technique. Is this medical procedure in any way relevant to the sorts of things we've been talking about, in terms of developing measurements of degrees of consciousness?

MM: Well, people have been trying to develop ways to ensure that patients who are undergoing anaesthesia are actually unconscious. Researchers have been developing devices that try to read from the brain and give an indication of consciousness for people who have been put in a medically-induced coma or placed under the influence of anaesthetics. So in a sense, people have been using those situations to address similar questions to those that I've been addressing. But aside from a study where I examined perfectly healthy people undergoing anaesthesia, there are naturally some different questions that they are asking that I have not been asking.

HB: Neurophysiologically-speaking, what is the difference between being in a coma and being under anaesthetics?

MM: From a brain function point of view, they're very similar. A very interesting paper came out about three or four years ago showing that from a brain function point of view, the two are almost identical.

Questions for Discussion:

1. Is the widespread applicability of mathematical thinking to the natural sciences a sign of the inherent mathematical order of nature or rather a reflection of the way humans think?

2. Can you give other examples of how a comprehensive theory of consciousness might be concretely applied to the medical realm?

X. Language and Thought

The Whorfian Hypothesis and Italian football?

HB: I'd like to turn now to another area of your research, the inter-relation between language and thought. This was something that was part of your doctoral work, you mentioned earlier, as well as being fundamentally related to issues that preoccupied you as an "orange-musing" child.

MM: Yes. I've always been very fascinated by language. Let me put it this way: humans have been thinking about this for a long time. Aristotle and Plato have clear positions on whether ideas exist in our brain or if we acquired them somehow.

More recently, people have been making a type of inference that goes along these lines: humans are extremely special in that there's no doubt that the ways by which we're manipulating our environment are very unlike most other species on the planet—sending rockets into space, installing satellites around the earth to enable people to communicate with each other even though they are thousands of miles apart, and so forth.

And some people associate these unique things that we can do with another unique aspect of our brain, which is language.

Other animals have some very elaborate communication systems, but no other species has language the way we do. Certainly no other species uses language in the particularly rich and profound ways that we use it. Other species use language in a very concrete way that has to do with their environment, safety and important social relations.

A lot of people wonder if the reason why we can do all these unique things is, at least in part, because our brain is very unique, with this unique linguistic capacity. People have been looking at this for, I would say, the last one hundred years throughout the domains of linguistics and psychology—and of course in philosophy for much longer than that. In the 1800s, people started contemplating the possible role of language as a formative aspect of our brain.

The argument was that the thoughts you have only arise because you speak a certain language. If you spoke a different language, your thoughts would be different.

This point of view is also usually associated with the following approach: you don't interact with the world directly. Rather, you interact with the world through your language. Just in the same way that the lenses in your eyes are a necessary interface between you and the world, in the same way language is your interface with the world and you organize the information that is coming to you from your senses in certain categories because that's the structure that your particular language gave you.

This argument is often referred to as the Whorfian Hypothesis. It literally asserts that you have the thoughts you have because you happen to speak a certain language.

Now other people, and I find myself in this other camp, think that we interact with the world through biology, our sensing organs, and then we use language to express the thoughts that our brain can have.

There is a very heated debate between these two views, but there's one particular aspect of this that has captured my interest, which concerns the notion of hierarchies.

One unique aspect of our brain is our ability to understand hierarchical dependencies: things that have structure, that have order. Just think of language: you can't just put words randomly one after the other and make a meaningful statement. The same is true with mathematics: you can't randomly put algebra and mathematical signs one after the other and create something meaningful. You can't randomly put notes one after the other and have a pleasing melody. They all have a certain structure.

So the question to me is: the structure that exists in math, in music, in logic, does it have any connection with the structures that we have in language?

HB: So, let me interject for a moment and back up a bit. There's a debate about whether our language is structured by our thoughts or whether our thoughts are structured by our language.

MM: Exactly.

HB: And my sense is that you are looking to probe matters more concretely by looking at, as you say, how the brain deals with hierarchy and structure in all sorts of different domains.

We'll get back to this shortly, but first I'd like to ask you a personal question. You are someone who is a native Italian speaker, although you speak English with great eloquence and fluency. Do you find that you have somewhat different thoughts, or could even be regarded as being to some extent a slightly different person, when you're speaking Italian as opposed to when you're speaking English? Or are you just Martin, translated into Italian, English or whatever else you happen to be speaking at the time?

MM: Well, when I swear during football matches, it naturally comes out as Italian. But short of that, my thoughts feel pretty similar. It never happens to me that I can think something in one language and can't think the same thing, or understand the same concept, in another.

HB: Well, OK, but that's a slightly different question. My question was, Do you *think* differently in one language as opposed to another?

MM: I do not feel any difference. Whether that is a trustworthy index of what is actually happening—

HB: Well, it's an answer to my question, which is all that you can reasonably do it seems to me.

The reason I'm asking you this is that, however subjective it may be, that strikes me as a concrete instantiation of one side of this particular coin. My sense is that you are effectively saying, "*I have all sorts of thoughts. These thoughts are independent of language, and then they come out—I express them—in whatever language I happen to be speaking at the time."*

In other words you are averring your personal belief in the notion that thought has primacy over the language.

MM: Exactly.

HB: Whereas the other view would be, "*No, no—I am actually somewhat of a different person somehow—the particular language somehow molds and effects my thoughts.*" So I've got your bias here.

MM: I should say that my bias here is data-related. I don't know if I went into this debate with a specific wish, one way or the other.

HB: Fair enough, you're an open minded individual, I never meant to claim anything to the contrary. Although it should probably be stated for completeness that it's possible that you had an a priori belief that naturally led you to interpret your own experiences—what you just referred to as "data"—in a particular way.

Questions for Discussion:

1. Is it possible, even in principle, for us to objectively evaluate the extent to which our language, culture and other associated personal historical factors, influence our thoughts?

2. Might enhanced neuroimaging techniques one day provide a clear and unequivocal "answer" to the Whorfian Hypothesis? (Readers interested in further exploring the Whorfian Hypothesis, sometimes called the Sapir-Whorf hypothesis, are referred to two other Ideas Roadshow conversations: **Babbling Barbarians** *with David Bellos and* **Speaking and Thinking** *with Victor Ferreira.)*

XI. Structural Similarities?

Comparing language, mathematics and music

HB: As you say, this is a debate that has gone on for a very long time, but my understanding is that you believe that by looking more closely at the structure of language, by looking at these hierarchies you were just speaking about, we might be able to quantify things more clearly. You make an analogy between arithmetic and the structure of language. Tell me more about that.

MM: Sure. A very simple example that I've used in a slightly more elaborate form is to look at the sentences "John kissed Mary" and "Mary kissed John". These two sentences have a similar relationship to "5-3" and "3-5".

Exactly the same tokens in each of these expressions have a certain position, and the specific position occupied allows us to infer meaning. Within each pair, the meanings are extremely different: who's the agent—who's kissing whom—and which number is getting subtracted from the other and so forth.

The question to me is, *The fact that we recognize this difference, the fact that we're sensitive to the position in which tokens appear in these expressions, is this a consequence of our ability for language?*

Does this ability in math, for example, this ability to understand the difference in meaning between 5-3 and 3-5, somehow *derive* from our ability for language?

We've actually tried to measure this empirically, by testing healthy volunteers. We put them in an fMRI machine and we took pictures of the metabolism of their brain while they were using their language faculties to understand the relationship between different tokens in a sentence; and we took pictures of their brain while they were solving similar problems, but now in math.

A simple example was the following: I could tell you, "*X gave Y to Z*" and then say, "*Z was given Y by X*" and ask you if these two phrases express the same state of affairs. You would reply that of course they do.

Then I could do something very similar in math. I could ask if "*X+Y is greater than Z*", is the same as "*Z-Y is smaller than X*". You would likely think about it for a bit, and then say yes.

In a sense, in both cases you're exercising the same type of syntactic sense that is applied here to language and there to math.

Now, the question is—at least the way we frame it—if our sense of syntax in math comes from the sense of syntax in language, we ought to see the *same* parts of the brain that you use to understand syntax in language be engaged when you're thinking of these related algebraic problems.

It turns out that that's not the case. The parts of your brain that you use for language naturally apply to language, but they do *not* get used for the similar task in the domain of algebra.

This was fairly surprising, but it conforms quite well with the data showing that aphasic patients whose language skills are so diminished that they can't identify the agent—who is doing the kissing in the phrase "John kissed Mary", say—can still do math pretty well.

HB: So they're using different parts of the brain in these two processes.

MM: That's right.

HB: More generally, what do you think these results imply about the debate we were discussing a moment ago about thought structuring language or language structuring thought? What sorts of conclusions or suggestions do you feel you can draw from your experiments?

MM: I've looked at this problem from several different points of view now: in math, in logic and now we're looking at it in music. It seems to me that language is somewhat insular. That is, language is a part of our brain, and it does language.

I almost find myself surprised that I have to say it. Nobody would think that the parts of your brain that you use for seeing were also those you would use for smelling. That would be strange. It's just not how our brain works.

The parts of our brain that we use for language are used for that and are very specialized for that. These other types of syntaxes or structures get worked out in very different parts of the brain.

HB: Have we done anything similar with other animals? You talk about language being particular to humans, but can we look at other members of the animal kingdom and think about ways of applying diagnostic techniques sort of like this?

MM: Absolutely, that is exactly the right question. I look at people who have language skills and math skills and see if the two are in a certain relationship.

Interesting questions include animals who don't have language the way we do—what capacities do they have, in math or in logic? It turns out that fish, for example, can do transitive inferences.

HB: No. *Fish?* Is this a particular type of fish? Some super-smart fish?

MM: Well, I must say that these transitive inferences that were studied were based on relationships of dominance, of hierarchy within a school, so that's something very relevant to them.

A fish can observe two other fish interacting—I imagine that in their brain they're working out who the dominant one is—and then, as a consequence, when they get put in the tank with one of these two fish, they know exactly where they belong in the hierarchy.

This is why we can say that it is a transitive inference—something like: *Bill is taller than Bob, Bob is taller than Mary, therefore Bill is taller than Mary.*

Some animals can make transitive inferences. A lot of animals can do pretty interesting things with math. They certainly can count with low numbers.

For example, you can display two boxes, one with two raisins in it and the other with one raisin in it. If you then cover up the boxes and transfer a raisin from one box to the other, they will now go to the box that has two. So they understand addition, so to speak.

You can go further still. If you have five raisins in one box and two in the other, and then move just one over from the box that had five in it, they will *still* go to the first box that has more raisins in it—that is, they opt for the one with 4 rather than 3. So at least with low numbers they can count, and there's some evidence that they can go beyond five or six, up to ten or more.

It's the same thing with young children who are prelinguistic—it's not quite right, actually, to say that they are prelinguistic, as they have the capability for language but are not yet able to express themselves linguistically.

But at any rate, these children can do similar tasks well before they begin to talk: they can appreciate addition and subtraction. They get surprised if you show them something that, mathematically doesn't seem to make sense—perhaps you have two objects and you pull one off and then you pull down a curtain and there are still two objects, they express surprise.

HB: Let me return for a moment to these ideas of language and thought. You're doing these experiments exploring syntactic structures by creating analogous expressions in arithmetic, and in logic, and in music. You're thinking about experiments that measure the brain activity in terms of the nested syntactic structure of language and a similar structure within music. What does that mean, exactly?

MM: If you ask someone who does music theory, they will say it has to do with patterns of tension and relaxation. For example, if you play a scale, you start with a C and then by the time you get to the B, you're sort of waiting anxiously to return to the C again. You have this relationship of expectation, which is no different than the type of expectation you form as someone is talking. You form expectations of possible transitions: what the next word might be, and so forth.

This led people to think that we might be building similar representations in music as we do in language. Linguists often build these upside-down trees where you start with a sentence that gets divided into several branches, and the way in which these branches connect expresses hierarchy.

For example, if I say "The dog barks", "the" and "dog" are connected to each other and the sum of these two connect to "barks". So it is not the same that in the sentence, "The dog barks", "The" and "dog" and "barks" are all on an equal footing. There is a certain hierarchical structure that places "the" and "dog" together.

Think of motor actions. If you want to eat something, you need to bring a spoon to a plate, and then the food to your mouth. It doesn't work in any other way. There's a hierarchical dependency there: the spoon has to go to the food *first* and *then* food and spoon must come to your mouth together. That's similar to language, in terms of "The dog barks". People make a similar argument concerning music.

One way to express this musically is by making sequences of musical chords and then suddenly violating the expected next chord. Then they see whether what happens at the point of violation is similar to what happens if I were to say something in a sentence that also upsets some expectation. So people have been looking at this.

We are looking at ways in which people produce different syntactic constructs in language—active and passive for example—and then explicitly comparing that to some analogous sense of syntactic structure in music.

Questions for Discussion:

1. To use the concepts invoked in an earlier chapter in this conversation, do you think that the example of fish making transitive inferences is more like an evolutionarily-bred reflex than a form of thinking or consciousness?

*2. Might it be possible that language and mathematics **are** structurally linked in terms of fundamental brain processing principles, but the particular instantiation of those activities happens in two largely distinct brain regions?*

XII. What Makes Us Human

In search of distinction

HB: Let me now ask you to speculate a little bit. It seems to me that we have two different scenarios.

One view is that people see language as the most important thing that separates us from other species: it's *the* distinguishing feature of mankind, it's a unique, high-level activity.

Then we have another view: that perhaps there is something more fundamental going on, and this syntactic structure, this nested structure, is just *one* manifestation of this. What really distinguishes humans is that we have this ability to form these high-level representative thoughts and ideas that can be expressed in, say, language, music and mathematics or logic or something else.

Would you be the sort of person who believes that second view, do you believe there is something particularly special about language per se, or do you believe something else entirely?

MM: I agree entirely with your second scenario. It seems to me that our mind has some property of understanding hierarchy and compositionality. These properties are expressed in several different ways. Language is maybe the most beautiful, the most obvious instantiation of these properties that we see most readily during the course of the day because we make so much use of language all the time. But to me it's just one instantiation of a more general functioning of the brain.

HB: So, it's just one mode—one mode of expression.

MM: Exactly. It turns out that this one mode is extremely representative of who we are, extremely embedded in being human. Language is such a deep part of being human. I'm not saying that language itself isn't amazing. I just don't think that language *itself* is the founding aspect upon which all these other things are built.

HB: So the thing that *is* the founding aspect, the kernel if you will, is that representative syntactic structure which manifests itself in different ways, one of which being language. Would that be a fair way to say it?

MM: Exactly. Our mind is completely symbolic, it's compositional, it understands hierarchies. And it shows these properties in all these beautiful ways, language being one of them.

HB: Very good. Thanks a lot Martin. That was a very enjoyable discussion.

MM: Thank you

Questions for Discussion:

1. Will we ever fully understand all the key organizational principles of the human brain?

2. To what extent will a detailed examination of the decision procedures of other animals enable us to better understand our own thought processes?

Beyond Mirror Neurons

A conversation with Greg Hickok

Introduction

Monkey See, Monkey Don't

In the late 1980s, neuroscientists at the University of Parma happened upon a discovery that many were later convinced had revolutionized our understanding of the brain: a certain group of neurons in the motor cortex of macaque monkeys were observed to respond not only when the macaque performed a certain action (grasping an object), but also when the monkey observed the experimenter doing so.

These neurons—eventually called "mirror neurons"—began to be implicated in a rapidly expanding list of theoretical constructs, not only for macaques, but also—rather more significantly—for humans. By the mid-2000s, mirror neurons were loudly trumpeted as instrumental to everything from language to empathy, while naturally providing, en route, an evolutionary bridge from macaques to humans.

Greg Hickok, a thoughtful and plain-speaking neuroscientist at UC Irvine, had first watched calmly from the sidelines as the mirror-neuron snowball swelled. As an expert in speech and language, Greg thought that the results were interesting, but well outside of his domain. By the early 2000s, however, growing numbers of advocates were maintaining that mirror neurons played a vital role in speech perception, and he felt compelled to react.

What was the proposed link between mirror neurons and speech and language?

"The mirror neuron cells in the macaque motor cortex were first found in a particular region called F5 (they were later found elsewhere

in the sensorimotor cortex as well), which was known to be the macaque homologue to Broca's area that has long been known to be a speech-related area in humans.

"Also lurking in the literature was an old theory called "the motor theory of speech perception" developed by Alvin Liberman, which said that we don't actually perceive the acoustics: the goal of perceiving speech is not to recover acoustic information but to recover the motor gestures that generated the acoustic signal.

"It was a reasonable, interesting, theory. And suddenly, you could put two and two together and say, 'Well, there's a psychological theory that says that we perceive speech in terms of recovering the motor gestures, and here you have macaque data showing that there are cells involved in responding to the perception of movements. Maybe this is the evolutionary precursor to what humans use for action understanding more generally, not just speech.'"

As Greg explains it, this interpretation does seems quite reasonable. The problem, however, is that experts in the realm of speech and language had long discredited the motor theory of language, recognizing that the perception and understanding of speech is actually quite unrelated to the motor system.

Many who had suffered damage to their frontal motor speech circuits and been diagnosed with a condition called Broca's aphasia, had significant disruptions to their ability to produce speech, but were able to understand it just fine. Meanwhile, conditions like cerebral palsy demonstrated that those who fail to develop a refined ability to control their speech articulators also have no problem with perception or understanding of speech.

*"There are, then, lots of situations that show that you don't need speech production abilities in order to perceive speech. **That** was why the motor theory was discredited. By the time mirror neurons were discovered, it was a dead theory in the mind of speech researchers.*

"But it was still lurking in the literature. So the neuroscience folks latched onto that without being aware of all the reasons why those of us in the language-speech domain had abandoned it."

Well, if mirror neurons aren't directly responsible for an underlying mechanism for language, what about focusing simply on the act of imitation?

Perhaps, goes the thinking, the ability to imitate enables us to establish a correspondence between ourselves and others that allows for empathy and the awareness of the mental states of others —so-called theory of mind—that, in turn, paves the way for meaningful societal interaction. And surely imitation must be a central aspect of the mirror neuron story? After all, when they were first discovered, mirror neurons used to be referred to as "monkey-see, monkey-do cells".

But it turns out that even imitation is much more complicated than might appear at first glance.

*"The reason people ended up **not** calling them monkey-see, monkey-do cells is that monkeys don't do that: they don't tend to imitate that way. And that was the big problem for that interpretation, because the obvious interpretation for these cells, if they're truly mirroring actions, is that they're the basis of imitation.*

"So the problem was that there wasn't a good behaviour in macaques that these cells could support."

Well, OK. So mirror neurons in macaques aren't responsible for imitation, because macaques don't really imitate in a significant way. But we do. So maybe the macaque mirror neuron system can be looked at as some sort of evolutionary forerunner to our own.

Perhaps. The difficulty there, of course, is that we are moving increasingly away from the original point of why people got so excited by the mirror neuron hypothesis to begin with. No longer the silver bullet to explain speech and language through the motor theory of speech perception, no longer a simple mechanism to explain a human-like imitation that macaques don't actually indulge in, we are left reaching for increasingly distant layers of speculation.

After all, even human imitation, however arrived at evolutionarily, is decidedly complicated. Clearly, imitation is a useful—indeed, vital—tool in our process of learning and discovery. But it's hardly the only thing going on. How do young children decide when to imitate and when not to? How can the neonate recognize that the tongue you're sticking out at her corresponds to the same sort of tiny pink object inside her own mouth? For imitation to work as a methodological learning tool, there must be something else going on.

> *"It has to be controlled by something. That really should be the target of what we're interested in understanding, not the simple mirroring or imitative mechanism itself."*

But if, more than 25 years after the original discovery, most of the core scientific mysteries remain intact, have we at least learned anything sociologically from the whole mirror neuron story, so that we might be less likely to fall prey to the next proposed cure-all that comes along?

> *"What I always tell my students to do, and what I always try to do, is read original sources. Often people just read review papers. For mirror neurons, there's a great one that came out in 2004. It's highly cited. For most people anxious to get the mirror neuron story, it's the one they read. But it's vital to recognize that all review papers are, necessarily, a synthesis—a rendering down of all the work that came before. You don't get the whole picture unless you read the original papers.*

> *"That's what I ended up doing with a group of students. We went back and read the original papers and realized that the story that had been rendered down to us was not supported by the prior evidence. I would suggest to any student who wants to understand something, go back and read the original reports and learn to spot assumptions and question every single one of them. Even in your own work. That's*

really important: to question everything that you do, and rethink things."

Imitation, in other words, will only get you so far. In science, like anything else, there's no substitute for the original.

The Conversation

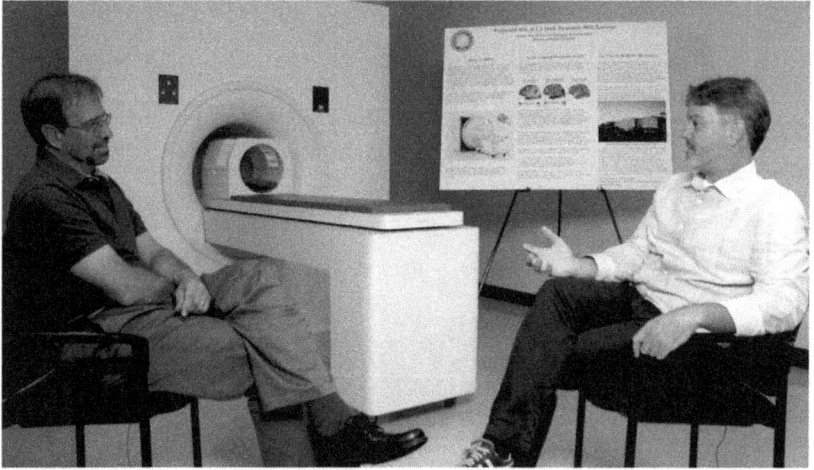

I. Talking Neuroscience

Speech, language and cognition

HB: How did your interest in cognitive science begin?

GH: I always liked psychology and was constantly fascinated by the mind. Through most of high school and the majority of my undergraduate education, I thought that I was on a clinical psychology track, going to do counselling of some sort. But once I started taking more specialized courses, I realized that I was much more interested in the neuroscience side than the clinical side. I remember being very stimulated by Oliver Sachs' book, *The Man Who Mistook His Wife for a Hat*. I was just fascinated by neurological disorders. I didn't know exactly what I wanted to do, but I knew I wanted to do something with the brain.

I also got involved in some research at the undergraduate level and I really enjoyed that. So it was those two things: being interested in the brain and interested in doing research—creating something new, discovering something new. That was very exciting for me.

I applied to a wide variety of experimental psychology programs where there was an opportunity to do brain-related research. I happened to get into one program where they were doing language and brain work at Brandeis University, and that's where I went—even though I wasn't particularly captivated by language at the time.

HB: What were your preferences back then?

GH: Well, like a lot of undergraduates, I was excited by the visual stuff: visual illusions and various things like that. The language part never excited me. I was always bored in the language sections of the Intro

Psych courses, because they would teach you what phonemes are, what morphemes are, what a sentence is; and that was just ridiculously boring for me.

But once I got into the program and started learning about language from a biological perspective, actually thinking of it in a different way, my interest grew. I started considering that language is essentially an adaptation of your brain that allows you to convert what you're thinking into wiggles in your mouth that can be communicated and implanted into someone else—which is a very different way to think about language. It became a biological question; and framed in those terms, it's much more interesting to me.

HB: I've talked to a fair number of people in the cognitive science field, and there seems to be this distinction—which is becoming, I suspect, ever blurrier—between those who say, "*I'm a behavioural person*," and those who maintain, "*I'm a biology person*". One indicator is that the biological guys will tend to use the word "mind" a lot, while the neuroscience guys will usually use "brain".

Did you feel that distinction when you were an undergraduate or graduate student? Did you feel yourself drifting to one side or the other?

GH: Well, the distinction still exists. There are people who do cognitive science and study the mind and don't care a lick about the brain: they explicitly say that it doesn't matter at all. Then there are people from the neuroscience side who say that we don't need to deal with cognitive theories or abstract constructs: all we really need is to dig into the neuroscience, and once we understand things at that level everything will be clear.

I've been exposed to both sides, and I find myself in the middle. I think that there are obvious benefits to both. It's really a linking problem. The psychological theories that have been developed in language and other domains are a description of real data. There are empirical facts, and there are abstract theories. We're not connecting it to neurons quite yet, but they are constructs that explain empirical data, just like in any science. And it's doing some work.

Meanwhile, in neuroscience you have information about, or data about information about, how information flows in the brain: what neurons do, how networks behave, and things like that.

The really difficult thing is trying to connect those two levels. That's where I see the most interesting direction for any of this sort of work.

HB: Are there increasing numbers of people trying to connect them? Or is the separation just growing wider?

GH: Well, the whole field of cognitive neuroscience, which is a relatively new term, is explicitly interested in connecting cognitive theories with the brain. But even within that you have people who value one sort of information over another in some cases.

A large number of people are explicitly trying to link cognitive theories with brain constructs. It was criticized quite a bit at the beginning, because it felt like neo-phrenology. People were doing these functional MRI experiments and pointing to areas that would activate while you were talking or thinking or doing whatever. They were calling it the speech area, the thinking area, or whatever.

Cognitive psychologists, rightly I think, criticized that work. Basically the critique was that just knowing *where* something happens in the brain doesn't tell you *how* it happens. And that's the critical question: how it happens. But as the field has matured, information about where things happen—what circuits are involved, what those circuits look like when we dig in a little bit more—is starting to inform cognitive theories quite a bit.

HB: As an outsider, it seems to me that an obvious difference between so-called neo-phrenology and old-fashioned phrenology is that now you actually have scientific devices that measure things, as opposed to some guy just feeling your head and guessing something about your character. I guess it's not quite that way, because back then they had some information from lesions and so forth, but for the most part, as you say, the difference now is that we have all this data. You can start modelling things more concretely.

But I've personally encountered a few people of what I would call an old-fashioned behaviouralist perspective who tend to be quite negative towards those who rely upon these modern diagnostic techniques for many of the reasons that you're saying, implying that, "*Well, it's all just collecting data basically. It's not actually building theories.*"

And it seems to me that, for the scientific enterprise to succeed, you need both.

GH: You do. The way I think about it is that when we first started doing brain-mapping with functional imaging, it was kind of like a big geography exercise: we're just mapping the landscape—which is kind of boring in some ways.

HB: But necessary.

GH: But necessary, yes. Once we get a lay of the land then we can start doing the geology: understanding how these things come about and what the forces are behind it. We're getting to the point where we're starting to do some serious geology.

HB: Let's get back to speech and language. You started off as a graduate student at Brandeis in speech and language, which was not an area of overwhelming desire for you at the very beginning. But then things started to change. What started getting you excited, and how did your research orientation develop from that point forwards?

GH: I actually started getting some education in formal linguistics and theoretical syntax, which—believe it or not—I found fascinating.

HB: Sure, I believe it. Why not?

GH: Well, a lot of people think, as I did when I first started, that formal linguistics is just philosophy. It's not a hard-core science.

HB: Well, I wouldn't say "just philosophy". That's demeaning to philosophy too.

GH: Yes, you're right. What I meant was that some people think that it's not an empirical science. But that's not true. The data are basically utterances generated by people who have the capacity for language. There are certain sorts of utterances that we do generate and others that we don't, for reasons that are not clear. Syntacticians are trying to understand what those principles are, and they're developing theories that can be tested by looking at more utterances. So it's an empirical science like any other.

It was fascinating to me how structured this system was, and it made me rethink something that was very human. Other animals don't seem to have language on this scale. Many of them communicate quite effectively, and in complex ways, but human language is unique in many aspects. Like I said, just being able to transplant an idea from one mind to another is a really interesting phenomenon.

So that got me very interested, and I actually started out doing psycholinguistics—just straight experimental psychology—even though I got into it because I was interested in the brain. I didn't do much neuroscience research as a graduate student. It wasn't until I went to MIT as a postdoc that I started doing a little bit more neuroscience. But this was all pre-fMRI, so we were limited to stroke patients and things like that. It was very different than it is today.

HB: And of course there's the big factor which is certainly implied in what you're saying: that language in and of itself is clearly hugely important as a distinguishing factor unique to humans. If you want to understand how the human brain is different from that of other animals, it's an obvious place to be looking. It may not be the only place to be looking, but it's certainly one very significant aspect.

GH: Right. Interestingly in the history of neuroscience and psychology, language has been used as a test case for theories of mind/brain over and over again.

It was a centrepiece in the debate over phrenology, or, more generally, whether you could localize different regions of the cortex in terms of different functions, which was the fundamental core idea in phrenology. Even though the pseudoscience of phrenology turned out to be incorrect in terms of measuring bumps on the head, the idea that different parts of the cortex were specialized for different things turned out to be true; and language was one domain that was testable for that.

One of the functions that Gall (Franz Joseph Gall, often claimed as the "founder of phrenology") had proposed is language. In fact, there's a story that that was the motivation for his theory in the first place. Apparently, he knew somebody who had very buggy eyes and was very loquacious, and he thought, "There must be a brain back there that's really developed, pushing on his eyes."

Then, throughout the 1800s, people were looking to language as the one function that was easily testable, as a way of seeing whether the different parts of the cortex were doing different things.

It came back in the 1950s and 1960s with the so-called "cognitive revolution", when behaviourism dominated American psychology. Then Chomsky pointed out that the structure of language is such that you can't explain it in terms of simple behavioural principles. So language has been used over and over again.

Questions for Discussion:

1. In what ways are the sociological divisions in contemporary cognitive science significantly different than other areas of science?

2. To what extent is it reasonable to have a theory of the mind without a detailed understanding of the brain?

II. Enter Mirror Neurons

Grasping monkeys and old theories

HB: I'd like to get back a little bit later on to the idea of localized function versus distributed function in terms of plasticity—hopefully at the end we can return to that. But, at least for part of this conversation, I'd like to talk about your book, *The Myth of Mirror Neurons*.

Before we start, though, I think it's worth highlighting something that you told me a few minutes ago, which was that the whole issue with mirror neurons was something that arose quite accidentally for you in the midst of your research activities.

You mention this in your book as well: how you had heard about these things in the course of your work and started getting asked questions about them at seminars. So you thought, *Okay, well, let's investigate this and find out what's going on.*

But it's probably worth emphasizing that one should not confuse Greg Hickok the cognitive scientist with Greg Hickok the mirror neuron critic. That's not all you do in life, and that's hardly the sum total of how you look at yourself as a researcher, either.

GH: Yes, absolutely. I got involved in mirror neuron research accidentally because I was studying sensory motor processes in speech, mostly from a motor control standpoint. We were noticing that the auditory system is deeply involved in controlling our ability to talk. You see this intuitively when you get a bad phone connection: if you get feedback that is out of sync with what you're saying that disrupts your ability to talk. That's because your auditory system is playing a really important role in generating speech.

We were studying this phenomenon and identified the relevant circuit in the brain using functional MRI. And we were beginning to investigate that in more detail when the mirror neuron discovery highlighted sensory motor function but in the reverse direction: the role of the motor system in perception. So we overlapped, essentially, in research interests, but with opposite perspectives. I was compelled to take the mirror neuron claims seriously and see what was behind them.

I first heard about mirror neurons in a lecture that Giacomo Rizzolatti gave—I think it was at the Cognitive Neuroscience Society meeting in San Francisco. It was fascinating. There were these cells that were responding both when the monkey was generating actions and observing actions, and everyone was interested. It was starting to gain some steam. That was back in the early 2000s, I believe.

But I ignored it. It wasn't relevant to my work at all. I had no interest in it. Even though the mirror neuron folks were claiming that it had relevance to speech, I knew it couldn't be the case, because of a condition known as Broca's aphasia.

It's been known since the 1860s that when you damage the frontal motor speech circuits, you can disrupt the ability to produce speech quite severely, while not necessarily impairing the ability to perceive or understand speech or language.

So I thought at that time that, while maybe the mirror neuron story held for monkeys and their actions; in terms of speech—my area of research—it just didn't pan out.

HB: I'm going to interrupt you for a moment, because we have to assume that not everybody knows the basic story of what Rizzolatti and his colleagues discovered with these monkeys.

My understanding is that these guys noticed—quite coincidentally when they were studying macaque monkeys for something else I believe—that the same neurons were firing when these monkeys were looking at someone else do a particular action —I believe it was grasping something—as when they were doing that action themselves.

GH: Right.

HB: And my recollection is that, because these neurons that are firing for both observation and action were in a particular part of the macaque's brain—the so-called F5 area that was considered to be roughly the equivalent of Broca's area in humans that is largely responsible for language and speech—people started going crazy with various hypotheses. Is that a fair summary of things?

GH: Yes, exactly. It's worth emphasizing that these cells were discovered in a context of a really beautiful research program that was directed by Rizzolatti involved in trying to understand how we control actions like grasping, generally.

They were interested in understanding how we use objects to shape information, to guide action. When you reach for something, you don't just blindly reach out and grope for it. You take the shape and the location of the object into account and shape your hand according to the object's size. So there's got to be a way to integrate that visual information with your grasp selection, essentially.

They were studying this with macaque monkeys. And, like you said, in between trials they were noticing that some of the cells in the monkey's brain that they were recording from responded not only when the monkey reached for things but also when the monkey observed the experimenter swapping out the objects between experiments.

That was fascinating, and hadn't been observed before in the motor cortex. Then the natural question was, "*How do you interpret this? What is going on?*"

The first, most obvious interpretation was that they were a kind of imitation cells: "monkey-see, monkey-do cells".

HB: Didn't you say that's what they were actually called for a while?

GH: Yes. Some people did call them monkey-see, monkey-do cells.

HB: That's a shame, I wish they would have kept going with that.

GH: Well, the reason they ended up not calling them that is because monkeys don't do that. They don't tend to imitate that way. And that was the big problem for that interpretation, because the obvious interpretation for these cells, if they're truly mirroring actions, is that they're the basis of imitation.

But it turns out that monkeys don't imitate in the same way that humans do. Right now, for example, we're copying each other's leg positions. That's quite typical of humans, actually, to mirror each other.

HB: Now I'm feeling self-conscious.

GH: I know.

But macaques don't do that. So the problem was that there wasn't a good behaviour in macaques that these cells could support. But they noticed that they were recording them in F5, as you mentioned, the homologue of Broca's area that has long been known to be a speech-related area in humans.

Also lurking in the literature was an old theory called "the motor theory of speech perception", developed at Yale University's Haskins Labs by Alvin Liberman and colleagues, which said that we don't actually perceive the acoustics: the goal of perceiving speech is not to recover acoustic information but to recover the motor gestures that generated the acoustic signal.

We don't need to go into the details of these claims, but it was a reasonable, interesting, theory. And suddenly you could put two and two together and say, "*Well, there's a psychological theory that says that we perceive speech in terms of recovering the motor gestures, and here you have macaque data showing that there are cells involved in responding to the perception of movements. Maybe this is the evolutionary precursor to what humans use for action understanding more generally, not just speech?*" And that was really the foundation of the theory.

The problem, though, is in the speech world, that theory had been discredited for reasons that I've already mentioned. We know that we don't need a motor-speech system to perceive and understand speech.

HB: Because those who had damaged that particular area of their brain were still clearly able to understand speech and language.

GH: Yes, exactly. This holds up from lots of different sources of data: from Broca's aphasia that I mentioned, which is the most obvious thing to look to, but also instances of cerebral palsy, where kids fail to develop the ability to control their speech articulators, but can perceive speech just fine.

There are, then, lots of situations that show that you don't need speech production abilities in order to perceive speech. That was why the motor theory was discredited. By the time mirror neurons were discovered, it was a dead theory in the mind of speech researchers.

But it was still lurking in the literature. So the neuroscience folks latched onto that without being aware of all of the reasons why those of us in the language-speech domain had abandoned it.

Questions for Discussion:

1. *Does the fact that mirror neuron researchers had unthinkingly "resurrected" an abandoned theory of speech provide a concrete instance of the dangers in sub-specialization of the scientific research community?*

2. *What do you suppose Greg means, exactly, by "action understanding"?*

3. *Are you surprised at the notion that, at least in some instances, humans imitate each other more than monkeys do?*

III. One Size Fits All?

The kitchen sink of cognitive science

HB: And it went even beyond that, I understand, into all sorts of bizarre areas where people started claiming that mirror neurons play a seminal role in the underlying mechanisms.

There's an interesting sociological aspect here to *The Myth of Mirror Neurons*, which I think can be decoupled and abstracted away from cognitive science per se, which is how theories become a panacea, the cure-all for everything. Suddenly they start being applied all over the place for every possible condition. How does that tipping point actually get reached? Perhaps we can talk about that a little bit later.

But for now let's mention some of the other areas. One area you certainly can see some sort of a plausible conceptual link to is empathy and autism.

GH: Right. The mirror neuron theory, like I said, was initially extrapolated most seriously to language. There was a follow-up paper to the major empirical reports in 1992–1996, which is when the monkey work was reported. A theory was proposed in '98 implicating language more seriously.

That was accompanied by another paper in '98 that talked about the ability of these cells to perform mind-reading operations, which isn't as crazy as it sounds. It's basically the idea that as humans we understand that our behaviour is controlled by our own mind, and that our minds are separate from other minds, and that your behaviour is controlled by your own beliefs, desires, and so on.

We call this the ability to mentalize; it's also called "theory of mind".

This, it has been argued, like language, is something fairly specific to humans. There are debates about that, but the general consensus is that it's another one of those big things that make us human. In this context, mind-reading is essentially the idea that if I'm trying to predict your behaviour, I look at your behaviour and make inferences about what you're thinking to try to read your mind.

HB: Based upon a correspondence with what you're thinking, and your experiences. You're able to project, as it were.

GH: Exactly. The basic idea is that, just like mirror neurons simulate movements that you're observing and allow you to understand them through simulation, we can read minds in the same way.

I see what you're doing, I can then simulate your mental state based on what I would do in a similar circumstance, which explains mind-reading in a fairly simple way. That was a big thing.

Empathy, you can see, would follow quite readily. The way I understand what you're feeling is by putting myself in your place, simulating what you're going through. Then I can *actually*, rather than cognitively, imagine what you're going through. I can *physically feel it* because I'm simulating what your situation is. You can see how that could explain empathy quite readily.

Imitation was something that was discussed, even though it doesn't exist as strongly in macaques, as I said early. Humans imitate a great deal. Some people have even called our species *homo imitans* for our prodigious ability to imitate and copy other members of our own species.

These are the sorts of things that were thought to be supported by the mirror neuron system in humans. Now it turns out that these are the sorts of abilities that people have claimed autistic individuals have difficulty with: mind-reading, language, imitation, empathy, and so on.

That led to the idea of the "broken mirror" hypothesis for autism. Which makes sense. All of this makes sense if you assume that mirror neurons are the basis of action understanding. With that foundation you can build fairly elaborate and logically reasonable theories.

HB: There are a couple of other things that are perhaps worth high-lighting. The first is on the experimental side. As you said, they were able to locate these mirror neurons in this particular part of the macaque brain: this F5 region, the homologue to Broca's region.

But during these experiments they actually had recorders that were picking up neural activity in the macaque brain. We haven't done these experiments with humans for all sorts of ethical and other reasons. So there's this outstanding empirical question, of, "*Well, do these things exist to the exact same degree in humans?*"

There was this inference that they were in the macaque brain, so therefore they must necessarily be in the human brain to a relatively similar extent. I think it's important to specify that it was impossible to perform the same experiments in exactly the same way to be able to determine that with any absolute level of precision for humans as well.

In fact, as I understand it, there were some pieces of evidence that were not completely in line with that hypothesis.

GH: A lot of the early work in humans was just documenting the existence of something like a mirror neuron system in humans.

That was the big question early on. Because if you could document it, and you had the interpretation of the monkey mirror neurons nailed down, then you could build these theories that we talked about. So a lot of work was really aimed at trying to determine whether these existed in humans by inference.

Although in general they were thought to be supportive, if you look closely these early attempts weren't all that supportive of the existence of mirror neurons in humans. For example, the first imaging experiments that Rizzolatti and colleagues tried in collaboration with other groups failed to show evidence in PET (positron emission tomography) studies of the overlap between action execution and observation.

They did see activation near and around Broca's area during observation, but they weren't the same areas that responded in both execution and observation. Later on Rizzolatti referred to this as a rather disappointing state of affairs.

It wasn't until 1999, when Marco Iacoboni showed that the same region of Broca's area in humans responded during the observation of actions, and the imitation of those same actions activated the same regions in Broca's area.

So the evidence was rather thin. Even that was problematic because the macaque mirror neurons don't seem to respond to imitation. So something different was happening in the human case.

A lot of people doubted whether these systems even existed in humans. I was never one of the doubters. If I ask you to copy a movement, you can do it. So there's got to be a way for you to take information you're seeing in my movements and regenerate them in your own motor system.

HB: Okay, but hang on. I can copy movements, I can do all sorts of things, but that doesn't necessarily mean I have neurons that are dedicated to copying.

I mean, there may be systems, there may be "copy systems" in my mind that do that. The idea that there are particular neurons that are necessarily lighting up when I see actions just as they would when I do actions, that doesn't seem to necessarily follow. All I know is that, empirically, I can copy movements.

GH: Right. It doesn't necessarily follow, but there has to be a way of connecting what you're seeing with what you're doing. So there's got to be some sort of a sensory motor system that's informing that mapping—whether they're individual cells tuned to seeing this and doing this, that's impossible to know at present.

But what we *do* know from the work that Rizzolatti and others have done on object-hand movement interaction is that when you are able to coordinate the perception of object shape with hand grasping, you would always find cells that responded to that shape with an appropriate hand-grasping action.

It would respond to an orange shape and some particular hand movement. Just by inference. To me, I didn't need to see the evidence. It just made sense that such a system would exist.

There's been general confirmation that these cells do exist. There was one study by a group in London that showed that there were regions in Broca's area that responded both to observing object-directed actions and generating those same actions. I think it was only ten participants, though—so, not a lot of data.

Then there was a group at UCLA that showed evidence in neuro-surgical patients. They recorded in individual neurons during clinical procedures while doing some research (with the subject's permission of course). They found evidence for cells that responded both during observation, and execution, of actions. They didn't record in Broca's area as far as I know, but I believe they found this in another motor area called the SMA.

HB: This brings up another point that I remember you making in *The Myth of Mirror Neurons*. If memory serves, you talk about how researchers had found mirror neuron systems in the parietal area (I think) of macaques, well outside of F5, and you remarked, "*Perhaps if they had actually found this system first people wouldn't have neces-sarily made that link with speech and language*".

Part of that jumping on to the full mirror-neuron hypothesis was the coincidence that they had first found these in a particular part of the macaque's brain.

GH: That's right. The circuit that they were studying—the so-called dorsal stream, or sensory motor circuit—includes area F5 in the sensorimotor cortex but also the parietal lobe areas, and the intrap-arietal sulcus. Both of those regions have been studied in terms of their sensory motor properties.

I do think that the fact that they discovered them in F5, which is thought to be the homologue of Broca's area, just called up the analogy with speech and the motor theory, and that led them down that particular path.

If they had found them first in PF, which is the parietal region where these cells are also found, it might have been linked to sensory motor processes, which is mostly what happens in the inferior parietal lobe in macaques, and things might have gone in a different direction.

Questions for Discussion:

1. What might be the evolutionary advantage of humans' prodigious ability, and tendency, to imitate?

2. How can Howard's concern about "systems vs. individual neurons" be rephrased using the concept of "reductionism"?

*3. Have you heard of "theory of mind" before this chapter? Those interested in a more rigorous treatment of this subject are referred to the Ideas Roadshow conversation **Exploring Autism** with Uta Frith.*

IV. Imitation

What it is and what it isn't

HB: I'd like to talk in some detail now about imitation. What are we really talking about here? Why do we care about imitation? What do we mean by imitation? Most of us naturally associate monkeys with imitation—there are these common expressions like "to ape something" or "monkey-see, monkey-do" or what have you.

When you look at the whole idea of imitation as a route to learning, to developing, to having more enhanced cognitive function, it seems that there are all sorts of interesting shades of grey that seem to come up along the way.

GH: Well, macaques don't seem to perform direct copying of the movements of others. Humans do it, but it doesn't seem to exist in macaques. But there are other forms of imitation. More broadly, imitation is something that seems to come in quite early in humans. There are some really heroic demonstrations of infants imitating in the neonatal wards.

HB: These are something like 42-minute old infants, if I remember correctly.

GH: Yes. They're doing tongue gestures—sticking their tongue out and pursing lips and stuff—and they seem to be able to copy.

HB: This is really fascinating to me. People actually did experiments with these hour-old children? They would go right into the maternity wards, and stick out their tongues or do whatever, and they would see that there was a statistically significant correlation with the infants doing that back to them.

GH: Yes that's right: there was. That led to the idea that imitation is innate, that it's something that humans are born with, this *homo imitans* idea.

HB: Otherwise it's a very productive first hour of life.

GH: That's right; you'd have to be learning really quickly—in the middle of the experiment, actually. So then the question was, *What does that do for you?*

The idea is that imitation provides the scaffolding for doing all sorts of things. For example, one idea is that once you have imitation you can build theory of mind: if I can imitate, that provides a correspondence, an innate correspondence, between myself and others, enabling me to understand the relation between my movements and your movements.

Then, through experience as I grow, I begin to realize that my movements are controlled by thoughts, desires, and wishes—I'm able to decide to move or not. And since I understand through my innate imitation ability that there's a correspondence between me and you, I can then make the inference that you have the same ability to control your own actions with your own mind, which is different from mine.

So that's the scaffolding for a really important thing in human cognition. There's been a lot of work on just trying to understand what exactly kids know in terms of their imitative abilities, and what they're capable of in terms of imitation.

According to some authors, then, theories of how language develops and how theory of mind develops are grounded in imitation abilities. There's a bit of controversy over that, but that was the critical point.

HB: And we all have this experience anecdotally. You see small children trying to learn a language, along with all sorts of things, and they're imitating constantly. They're imitating speech patterns, they're imitating words, they're imitating physical actions either at play or to get a better comprehension of what's actually going on. It seems like a pivotal aspect of the learning process.

But then you highlight two aspects of this—perhaps more than two, in fact, but two stand out in my mind—that are important and often overlooked subtleties.

First, there's this notion of correspondence: a 42-minute-old baby sees someone lean over and stick out his tongue and the baby responds in kind by sticking out its tongue. Well, we naturally assume that they can mimic, so we imagine that they are thinking something like, *Okay, he's sticking out his tongue, so I'm going to stick out my tongue back at them.* And we focus on questions like, *Can they perceive whether the tongue is being stuck out? Do they have the motor facility to be able to stick out their own tongue?*

But we're begging an awfully big question here, which is whether they're able to identify that *that particular thing* which is coming at them is the same thing that they have themselves.

We have to be careful and not assume too much. We should be able to distinguish between the motor capacities and the awareness, the visual capacities, and also this correspondence, being able to make this link. And you stress that this is both a fundamental issue and an easy one to overlook.

GH: That's been one of the main problems with understanding how we imitate, especially in those early studies. *How does the neonate know that the little thing coming out of that oblong-shaped object that they're looking at corresponds to some motor program that they can activate in their own brain to stick their tongue out too?* They've never seen their tongue. How do they know the relation?

HB: That's a huge jump.

GH: It is; and that's why the notion of "innate imitation" was important to get a lot of this stuff off the ground. If it's innate, then you don't have to worry about the correspondence problem. It's solved already. Through evolution.

HB: Well, it's solved structurally, in terms of its being axiomatic. But that doesn't tell you what's going on.

GH: It doesn't, no.

HB: I mean, we'll talk about mechanisms shortly, but that's the obvious question, isn't it? *What the heck is going on inside?*

GH: Exactly. Mirror neurons actually provide a potential answer, if the idea is right, in the sense that if mirror neurons evolved to support imitation, then they can be the mechanism that allows all of this to happen.

Even if the action understanding theory was incorrect, as I've suggested it is based on the sorts of stuff we talked about, mirror neurons could still be critically important for human behaviour if they supported imitation. Because imitation is, according to some, what gives rise to language and theory of mind.

Maybe that leads to empathy, and you can build the whole story on imitation instead of action-understanding. It's an important piece of the story.

The difficulty is that no one seems to believe that mirror neurons, at least in macaques, have anything to do with imitation. Rizzolatti has said that they don't support imitation in macaques.

And other researchers who study imitation, people like Andy Meltzoff at the University of Washington, are interested in mirror neurons because they look like imitation cells, but they've declared that they're obviously not enough to support imitation.

So the simple beauty of the mirror neuron mechanism, its simplicity, isn't enough even to explain imitation, which it looks like they're exquisitely designed to do. That's a problem. The usual story is that what happened is that mirror neurons in macaques evolved to support imitation.

But then you have to wonder what exactly evolved when you've got the mechanism built in. Then the question is whether it was the mirror neuron mechanism that evolved, or if it was the cognitive capacity to take advantage of that mechanism—to put it to use for whatever higher level behaviours you're interested in doing, like language—was what evolved.

HB: Because at some level we know, objectively, that there's a difference. Even if we've never heard of mirror neurons, we know that humans can do something that macaques can't, namely this special type of imitation: this knowledge-gaining imitation, learning imitation, or whatever you want to call it. We already knew that.

So the question is, *What's responsible for it?* If you posit that it's mirror neurons, because we see mirror neurons in the macaques—that alone, even if you assume that humans have the exact same mirror neurons, is no explanation.

Then you have to start positing something like "it's an enhanced mirror neuron that does that". But that's just tautological: that's just saying that it's a different structure, because the old mirror neuron system wasn't good enough to do that for you.

GH: Right, yes.

HB: The other thing that I think you're wonderfully explicit about saying in your analysis is that however beneficial imitation is, broadly defined or specifically defined, it's not the answer to everything in the educational world as it were.

You give a very concrete example of language acquisition, which I found to be quite telling, where you focus on a certain abstract level of generalizing that occurs "on top" of imitation, as it were.

You talk about how children never hear adults say "runned" and "goed" when they're speaking English, and yet they do come up with those sorts of things themselves. So they are imitating, but they're not *just* imitating: there is this process of generalizing, or invoking some level of abstraction, that they're doing. They're trying to fit patterns

This leads to this idea that imitation—however significant it is and however it may be linked to a mirror neuron structure or something like that system—is *but one aspect* of this learning process. It is not the end result nor is it necessarily the be-all-and-end-all of learning. Is that a fair way to say it?

GH: Yes, it is; and it's been something that's been worked out in speech language areas quite a bit. It's been suggested that we learn language by imitation: we just copy our parents. But if you look closely, even if you just scratch the surface, you realize that can't be the answer. Because, like you said, kids do things that aren't in the environment. They say things that they never hear. And they don't say things that they very well could imitate.

Suppose you didn't know English that well and you were interested in deriving appropriate questions from sentences. "*I saw Mary with John*" would be naturally paired with "*Who did you see Mary with?*" Now, suppose I said "*I saw Mary and John*". A natural analogous structure to that you might generalize to is, "*Who did you see Mary and?*"

But you don't do that. And kids don't do that. So there's something else going on: it's not just imitation. There's something a little more structured that tells kids, or their language system, what kind of things are part of their mental capacity for generating and understanding speech and language.

Questions for Discussion:

1. What does Howard mean, exactly, when he says, "But that's just tautological"?

2. Do children learn language differently than adults? If so, how much of that difference do you think is related to their use of imitation?

V. Seeking a Controller

Structural investigations

HB: OK, let me try to summarize your argument with respect to this question of imitation. Tell me if I've understood it correctly.

Imitation is an essential tool, an essential aspect, perhaps an essential by-product, of many of these learning processes that we have. But by ascribing to it the status of a driving force, or to be saying that at some level it's necessarily an end in itself, we're making the classic mistake of confusing correlation with causality.

Imitation may be an essential *part* of the learning process, it may even be a necessary *by-product*, to the extent that for humans, whenever there is learning going on, there is going to be some level of imitation involved.

But that doesn't necessarily imply that whenever you have imitation you're going to have learning; and therefore what we really need to focus on is the underlying structure to which this imitation is associated.

Is that a reasonable summary?

GH: Yes. Cecilia Heyes has pointed out that the mechanism for imitation is very simple: it's just an associative mechanism. You take some stimulus, some action, and you map it on to a motor program that can regenerate that. It's not a complicated thing. It exists in macaques. They have this fundamental ability in terms of the neural circuits, but they don't seem to take advantage of it.

Given that it's a simple mechanism, the question is, *How do you ramp it up to be really useful for you?* That comes down to the kinds of systems that can put it into play. It's telling that imitation as it exists in humans is very smart. Some of the work in kids suggests that they will imitate quite readily, but they *know* what to imitate.

If you try to demonstrate the operation of a novel toy, but you keep failing, the kid won't imitate the failure. That would be a direct imitation, a stupid imitation. They see what you're trying to do, make inferences about what the goals are, and then they imitate the successful way of doing it, even if they wouldn't have been able to know how to do it before.

HB: Right. So this is my sense of it being a tool. There has to be some meta-structure underneath, or over, or whatever.

GH: Yes, there has to be something driving it. Even in overt, unconscious imitation, which humans do—the leg-crossing copying stuff, which is called the chameleon effect—even *that* is smart. You can set up experiments where you put people in situations and have a model crossing her legs or scratching her head and people will tend to copy that unconsciously. But we don't do it willy-nilly. We tend to copy only people we want to identify with. If there's someone we don't like, we don't copy them.

So in that case there's something social behind the tendency even to unconsciously imitate. It's not just that simple associative mechanism that is allowing this system, the higher-level stuff, to develop. It's the higher-level stuff that's taking advantage of the simple mechanisms.

HB: Listening to you talk, though, I'm thinking that there are a few exceptions. The obvious thing that comes to my mind is yawning. This is something that we don't, for the most part, consciously do. Might this be looked at as some kind of a remnant of this underlying mechanism, some flaw that we're on the evolutionary road towards getting rid of at some point?

GH: Yes, mirror neurons have been implicated, at least speculatively, in contagious yawning. It seems to occur in animals as well, I believe.

I haven't thought deeply about it either, so I don't have a good answer for you.

But I do know that there is a tendency to imitate that we're constantly suppressing. It shows up in neurological disorders sometimes, and it's called echophenomena—echolalia in speech. With certain types of brain damage individuals will tend to repeat back what they hear. That's obviously not neurologically normal.

It's the same with imitating movements and actions. There are some cases where you can get people who just copy everything you do. That's an implementation of that simple imitative mechanism. But obviously if you really, literally, imitated everything everyone did, that would just be creepy. It's not normal.

HB: Sure. And not terribly efficient or productive, or any of that.

GH: No. It has to be controlled by something. That really should be the target of what we're interested in understanding, not the simple mirroring or imitative mechanism itself.

Questions for Discussion:

1. Do you think that the fact that "contagious yawning" also appears in other animals amounts to some measure of evidence of its "evolutionary advantage"? If so, what do you think that might be, exactly?

2. Why does Howard say, in his summary, that "we're making the classic mistake of confusing correlation with causality"? What does he mean, precisely, by this?

VI. The Community Responds

Sceptics and believers

HB: Let's move now to the issue of the scientific community's responses to your criticisms of the mirror neuron hypothesis.

I'm not a cognitive scientist, and I'm talking to you, so maybe you're just a particularly persuasive person. But I've read your book and I think, *Okay, this all seems to make sense to me. I get what this guy's saying.*

Clearly, as we've discussed, there has to be a physiological mechanism for imitation. Imitation is a very important tool but, in and of itself, it doesn't really solve these fundamental questions, including this correspondence problem that you specifically highlight.

So all of that seems very reasonable to me. Is everybody else in the community saying, "*This seems perfectly reasonable—this Hickok guy is right. We **did** get carried away, all of us...*"—or not?

GH: I don't know. I hadn't studied imitation all that much before writing this book. I knew it was something I had to deal with in this book for the reasons we talked about. It was important. It seemed relevant to mirror neurons. It was claimed to be a function of mirror neurons in humans, but not in macaques.

So I dug into it, and looked into all this literature about human imitation. It's fascinating literature. Kids are really good at it, there's no doubt about it. We obviously imitate, or learn a lot from imitating others. We watch what other people do and figure out how to do things. A lot of other species do the same thing, from dogs to octopus.

HB: Really? Octopus?

GH: Lots of other animals can do it. We call it "observational learn-ing", and it's been demonstrated in a range of species. There was an impressive demonstration of an octopus learning how to get into a container from watching another animal who had figured it out. It made headline news a couple of decades ago, I think.

So that ability is obviously important. But the claim that the ability to imitate generally is the basis for all of the things that humans can do, is something that I wonder about, and something that I haven't really talked about much publicly or written about except in this book.

But it seems to me that the story is a bit backwards based on what people are saying. I don't think imitation can be the foundation.

HB: It's a consequence.

GH: Yes, it's a consequence. It's something that a lot of animals can do, but humans have gotten really good at making use of it. I think that's because we've got other systems that know what to do with it. But I don't know how the field is going to respond to these ideas.

HB: Well, you must know a little. You've come out with this book recently; you must have had some feedback.

During our conversation you've given me a very compelling précis of things. But what I'd really like to know now is what those on the other side might be feeling.

GH: What I don't know is how the people in the imitation world will respond to my ideas about imitation generally. As far as the mirror neuron stuff, I know much better about how people will respond.

HB: But the ideas on imitation are part of a more general argument.

GH: That's right. As far as mirror neurons go, I was always a doubter, because my knowledge of the speech world suggested that the original mirror neuron theory just didn't pan out, and I was not sure it would pan out anywhere if it didn't work in speech. But when I started looking into it more seriously, I realized how weak the arguments were, and how weak the empirical evidence was—how circular their claims were in some cases.

When I started going public with my concerns, people would come up to me and say, *"You know, I didn't think they were doing what they said they were doing but now I realize that there's some truth behind my hunch."* So a lot of people came out of the woodwork, at least it seemed to me, as being doubters of mirror neurons doing what they were claimed to do.

What I found is that, if you believe in mirror neurons, if you are fundamentally convinced that they're involved in action understanding and that they generalize to everything else—and there are still people who are responding to my book online and by Twitter and my blog and things like that who really want to believe that mirror neurons do what they're claimed to do—it's very hard to be convinced otherwise. Their general response has been that I must be mistaken somehow, that there are other explanations for the kinds of problems that I brought up.

That's for the hard-core believers. Meanwhile, there's a large group of people who have a moderate view of mirror neurons. What I've mostly attacked in the book, and suggested alternative interpretations for, is the idea that mirror neurons support and form the basis of action understanding—that that's how we understand, through this simulation mechanism.

There are other people—including some of the folks who were involved in some of the early theoretical developments, like Michael Arbib—who have suggested a more moderate view, which is that mirror neurons aren't the basis of understanding, but they assist: they provide some sort of a supplemental boost to understanding.

HB: But that seems to me to be the same sort of notion as what we were talking about earlier regarding imitation: that it's a tool, a consequence of underlying cognitive processes, for human learning and understanding. It's *one* of the tools—maybe even a *primary* tool—that we use. And mirror neurons themselves are likely implicated in some way, broadly defined, as a key part of this imitation process. So we naturally have to pay attention to imitation—and, consequently, mirror neurons—to better understand and appreciate imitation, which is one aspect of the underlying structure of these fundamental cognitive processes.

Isn't that what we're talking about here? You're not saying that it's useless, or garbage, or irrelevant. And when you talk about action understanding, my sense is that you're focused on this underlying structure, right?

GH: Right. So maybe this is a good time to say what I think is going with mirror neurons. Then we can talk about how other people slightly differ from that view.

Questions for Discussion:

1. What do you think makes someone a "hard core believer" in a particular theory or interpretation? Is the disposition to being a "hard core believer" independent of the particular theory in question? To what degree is it reinforced by the prevailing social structures?

2. To what extent does the fact that Greg's research was well removed from many scientific aspects associated with the mirror neuron hypothesis make him an ideal person to objectively critique it?

VII. A Different Perspective

Prediction and sensory states

GH: I think that, in terms of processing actions, mirror neurons are doing exactly what these other neurons are doing for guiding hand movements or grasping objects on the basis of shape. The basic idea with object shapes is that you have visual information about these objects that allows you to select from your vocabulary, as Rizzolatti put it, possible grasps that you might use. It's basically a mechanism.

The integration of the visual information with the movement control system is one that allows you to guide actions or select appropriate actions. I think exactly the same is happening with mirror neurons. This is a circuit that is designed, or just developed through experience, to take not "object information" but "action information" of other animals, and use that to guide action selection.

Some of them happen to be mirror-related. In the case of humans, if I stick my hand out, that will tend to elicit a mirror-like response from you. That would involve the mirror circuit, I would say. But other actions I might engage in, like throwing a punch at your face, would elicit a different response. You're going to want to duck or do something else.

Basically, it's a generalized circuit that's involved in taking sensory information of a variety of sorts and using that to select appropriate actions, some of which happen to be mirror-like. They just keyed in on those. In fact, if you look at the early experiments, not all the cells that responded to perception as well as execution were mirror. There were some that were anti-mirror in fact.

HB: And they would have to be, from an evolutionary argument.

GH: Exactly. I think of them just like the normal circuit: nothing special. And just like these object-oriented cells are not involved in object understanding, the mirror neuron cells are also not involved in action understanding.

There's an interesting argument that is actually quite reasonable that comes out of the motor control literature.

The basic idea is that when we generate movements, we're regularly simulating, from the motor control perspective, that movement, neurally. This is referred to as an internal model.

As you're reaching for something, you generate predictions as to where your arm should be, which you can then confirm with somatosensory or visual feedback, to help control the movement. You're basically checking how far off from your prediction you are.

That's been fairly convincingly demonstrated as a mechanism that the brain uses. It's sometimes referred to as "forward prediction" or "forward control processes".

If that's the case, if generating movements is actually resulting in sensory modulation—modulation in the sensory cortex in terms of what you might predict—then you might use this mirror mechanism to predict the outcomes of people's movements. The basic idea is this: if I see you reaching for something, I can simulate that in my motor system, generating the normal forward prediction in my brain, predicting the sensory consequences which I can then use to process the information that's coming in on the sensory side.

It's not so much an understanding mechanism, it's more about predictive coding. I'm trying to figure out what's going to happen next in your movements.

I've actually proposed that something similar to that is happening in speech, which could explain some of the small effects that people see in terms of how stimulating the motor system results in a slight modification of how speech sounds are perceived—although I actually doubt some of my own claims now; I'm not so sure that that's even the case, for reasons that I talk about in the book.

But the point is that there are other ways of thinking about this system, and how it might augment perception, rather than necessarily be the basis of understanding. And our lab, together with many others, is exploring whether such a mechanism might assist.

HB: One thing that occurs to me, and perhaps this is just my own bias, but when I watch tennis players playing tennis, say, there are different ways of watching. If I watch closely and effortfully, I actually feel that I'm learning at some level.

This is a fairly known phenomenon, I think, which tends to work best when one watches an incredibly graceful athlete, like Roger Federer, play. When you focus on it, it's almost like you feel like you're playing yourself.

Now my sense is there is something going on in the learning process, just like when children are mimicking, or what have you. That's something that can be captured, and that's something that, with effort, you can presumably train to some extent; but I'm guessing there's a huge amount of complex mechanistic stuff that's underlying all of this.

GH: That's essentially a form of observational learning. You're able to take information that you're seeing and apply it in your own motor system or apply it to your own sensory motor system. Once you realize that you can take advantage of that, or once you have the ability—and lots of species do have the ability to do this—you can make use of it.

The sense that you get that you're actually doing the actions you're observing probably comes from something like the mirror mechanism, where you're able to simulate the actions. You activate the movements in your sensory motor system.

The critical thing is that it's not just the movements that are driving it. Any time you generate some action, you're generating sensory consequences to that action. As you practice your swing, you're not just generating movements. You are feeling the consequences, you're seeing where the ball hit.

The learning isn't just, as the mirror neuron people claim, in the motor system. It's feeling and recognizing the sensory consequences of that. What you really want to do is not just generate a particular movement: what you really want to do is see that ball land in the spot that you wanted it to land. You want the swing to *feel* right. You want the contact with the ball to have the right feeling, and you can do that with a lot of different movement patterns.

But your target, as with any movement—and this is the key—is really a sensory state. We're aiming for a sensory state. That's true in tennis, and it's true in speech. When you move your mouth you're not trying to implement a particular motor pattern. You're trying to generate a sound: that is, reproduce the sounds of the language that you've learned perceptually.

That's a really important distinction to make in what we're talking about here: the goals of movements are not the movements themselves, they're sensory states.

Questions for Discussion:

1. What, exactly, does Greg mean when he distinguishes between "object information" and "action information"?

*2. How would you describe the "internal model" hypothesis Greg mentions in this chapter in your own words? For additional background and perspectives on how our brains are regularly predicting, see **Minds and Machines**, the Ideas Roadshow conversation with Duke University neuroscientist Miguel Nicolelis.*

3. How do the "visualization techniques" of sports psychologists support Greg's claims that the goals of movements are sensory states?

VIII. Sociological Explorations

The merits of primary sources

HB: I'd like to plunge in a bit more deeply into the sociology of science now. The mirror neuron craze, which for at least some time was running rampant through the cognitive science community to the extent that it seemed like it was the magic pill for just about every possible concern, is that something that you've seen before in other guises? Do you say, *"Oh yes, I remember that. Now it's mirror neurons. Before that there was something else the last decade, and next decade there'll be something else"*? Or do you think it's a somewhat unique phenomenon?

GH: We always see fads in science. In my own scientific career I remember a lot of interest in *connectionist modelling*: a computer-based association, neural network-type modelling for human cognition. They were applying it to everything, and it got very popular. That's died down a little bit now. People still use it, but it's, shall we say, in its proper place now: it's useful, but there's an appreciation that it's not the answer to everything.

Before that, we could probably go back to the idea that everything could be solved in terms of symbolic logic and artificial intelligence computation. People were excited about that. Before that, I suppose, there was behaviourism: everything could be explained in terms of simple stimulus-response or operant conditioning and so forth.

I don't think this is anything terribly different than we've seen in the past. Like all of these previous fads, they get vetted in the scientific community. Those who are devout believers will push the idea as far as they can, while doubters, like me, will push back. We end up somewhere in the middle, usually, and it finds its rightful place. People move on.

I don't think this is particularly unique in that sense. In a broader sense, I suppose what's been special about mirror neurons, as opposed to some of these other crazes, is that their reach was so broad: seeking to explain everything from language to empathy so that it really looked like a revolution in explaining how the mind works while providing an evolutionary mechanism for it.

People talk about language and theory of mind and all these human things, but then explaining how it emerged has always been a problem. Connecting it to brain circuits—how the brain actually does this—has always been difficult, especially in cases where we don't have nice animal models where we can study the response of single units.

Mirror neurons seemed to provide all of that. They explained everything. There was a simple neurophysiological mechanism that you could point to that was the basis of it. It existed in a primate that was reasonably close to us, so that we could talk about common ancestors and how things might have evolved. It was the complete package in terms of explaining how the mind worked for a lot of human things. I think that's why it got so many people really excited.

HB: Is there anything we can take away, sociologically, from this? Let me be more specific. As a university professor, you're regularly involved with undergraduates, graduate students, postdocs, and so forth—many young people.

Granted that there is this inherent cyclical tendency for things to become all the rage and then, as you say, go into their proper place, is there some more concrete message that we can pass on to younger people?

Does it just boil down to fairly anodyne phrases like *Think more critically?* or *Don't believe everything you hear?* or can we be a little bit more specific?

GH: What I always tell my students to do, and what I always try to do, is read original sources. Often people just read review papers.

For mirror neurons, there's a great one that came out in 2004 ("The mirror-neuron system" by G. Rizzolatti and L. Criaghero). It's highly cited. For most people anxious to get the mirror neuron story, it's the one they read.

But it's vital to recognize that all review papers are, necessarily, a synthesis—a rendering down of all the work that came before. You don't get the whole picture unless you read the original papers.

That's what I ended up doing with a group of students. We went back and read the original papers and realized that the story that had been rendered down to us was not supported by the prior evidence.

I would suggest to any student who wants to understand something: go back and read the original reports and learn to spot assumptions and question every single one of them. Even in your own work. That's really important, to question everything that you do, and rethink things.

HB: Because this is not just a synthesis. This is the synthesis by someone who's an advocate of this particular perspective. That's normal, of course: you would expect the advocates to be doing the synthesizing—who has the time to bother synthesizing something she doesn't actually believe in?

But, of course, if you're listening to someone who believes fervently in Case A giving a synthesis of the arguments for Case A, it's worth bearing in mind that he's inherently biased. He's inherently non-objective. But I imagine that it's sometimes hard to keep doing that, and it's hard to not rely on syntheses, because everybody's busy and all too often one has to depend on others to synthesize things for you.

GH: Yes. I think that's why the mirror neuron enterprise went as long as it did. There was so much being generated, and it was so difficult to go back and look critically at everything. People were naturally doubting things, but they didn't have the time to go back and work out the details of why this was a problem.

It just takes someone who is motivated for whatever reason to go back and do that, to lay it out so that there's a new synthesis, or a counter-synthesis, that can point out what the problems are or at least what the alternative hypotheses are so that we can have some balance.

I think that's the way science works. We're all biased. I mean, I'm certainly biased to believe my own work. If I do an experiment and get a result, I believe it. If someone else gets the same result, I'm going to question it a little more. That's normal.

HB: But if you didn't believe what you were doing you wouldn't be in the business that you're in. We all believe in what we're doing. But we also recognize that there has to be an objectively compelling argument for it.

GH: Right. I see it in the perspective of an evolution of scientific ideas. People throw out all sorts of ideas that are reasonable. Not all of them are right: some of them are closer approximations to the so-called truth than others, and then they get debated. The fittest survive and persist; and the ones that are most valid, I suppose, are the ones that survive all of these fads and show up in all areas, essentially.

HB: I was right with you until you said, "the so-called truth". Are you not a realist? Do you not believe that we're actually converging upon some truth that's out there?

GH: Oh, yes. I do believe that.

HB: Because if you don't, we'd have to start all over again.

GH: Right. No, I do. That was a covert reference to some ideas that are being developed in terms of whether or not what we perceive in the world is actually veridical, or whether it's just an interface that allows us to operate. But that's a different topic.

HB: Sure, but there's something out there whether we can directly perceive it or not, I'm guessing you believe. You're not an anti-realist are you?

GH: No, no. I'm basically a realist.

HB: Hmm, "basically." All these weasel words, all of a sudden…

Questions for Discussion:

1. Are you surprised at the notion that science is subjected to fads and fashions like many other activities?

2. Should scientific journals make more of an effort to commission review articles from more "objective" quarters? What are some of the logistic challenges associated with that approach?

IX. Neuroplasticity

Speculations on the underlying mechanisms

HB: Earlier in our conversation, when we were talking about phrenology, we touched on the question of localized versus distributed brain function together with associated issues of neuroplasticity.

This sort of thing comes up in a lot of my conversations with cognitive scientists and it also came up in your book. People invoke this principle of "use it or lose it" as a way of looking at the evolution or the modification of the human brain. The notion that individual neurons and groups of neurons can change their function depending on their use seems to be fairly well-established these days throughout the neuroscience community.

I'm not questioning these results, and I understand that neuroscientists have seen evidence of this all over the place now. But I'm trying to understand what's going on, and I'm looking at a possible mechanism. And I find it confusing.

At first it seems very reasonable. Well, you have these things that the brain is hardwired to do, or at least has a potential to do, and then for whatever reason you're not using things in the usual way and so the natural functionality in that part of the brain switches to focus on something else that is also needed.

But when I actually think a little more about this, I don't actually understand it at all. Because there's a certain sense that there must be some kind of a threshold. At what point can a neuron switch from one use to another? That seems like it entails an entirely different structure. Maybe I'm not being very coherent here. Do you understand what I'm getting at here?

GH: I think so.

HB: The idea seems to be that the neurons that would have been used to do one thing are now doing something else, because they somehow can't do the original thing—we have some dysfunction or something that is stopping them from being used in the normal way, and so instead of being dormant, they switch to doing other things.

In a handwavy way I think, well, that makes sense—it's surely evolutionarily advantageous to be able to adapt like that. But then I ask myself, what's *actually* going on? At what point do these neurons decide that they're dormant? How do you even define *dormancy*? Is it once a month, once a year? It seems that you would somehow need to have this whole threshold mechanism associated with that notion of plasticity. Do you guys talk about that stuff?

GH: Yes. People who study plasticity are worried quite a bit about that. I don't study plasticity much but I'm aware of some of the issues, and I think I understand what you're asking.

One of the very clear demonstrations of plasticity on a low level is where, for example, if you were to remove a digit, and the part of your somatosensory cortex that was responding to the touch of that digit will tend to start to respond to touch of another digit. Basically the surrounding areas will take over that tissue.

So the question is, *What's actually going on there? How does it take over? What is the cell doing?* I think one answer to your question is that individual neurons are just doing what they do. They fire or not depending on the input. So there's nothing special about the actual function of the individual neurons that makes it tied to touch from this finger. It responds to touch from this finger because it's wired up to the nerves in this finger.

So how does it start responding to these things to say, "*Hey, I'm free. Anyone?*" Probably what's going on, and this is semi-speculation on my part (I have to go to the literature and check), is that there are already connections, cross-connections, and some projections from nerve cells here into the cortex that's responding to this. It's not a clean division.

HB: It's not a one-to-one map.

GH: Right. It's graded; and it mostly responds to one thing. But there are also some inputs coming from other fingers. Maybe what happens is when this digit goes away, these inputs from other fingers are the only things that are left. They start driving it, and pretty soon those synapses strengthen and you start getting responses.

So you get plasticity from connections that are probably already existing, connections that simply take over when the normal inputs that are driving an area aren't responding anymore. What people are seeing more and more is that where we thought an individual area was only getting input from one system, it's getting input from a lot of different systems.

HB: That's what I was going to ask. With fingers, you might be able to say, "*Okay, that's roughly the same area*", but more generally, are there restrictions due to localization of processing?

GH: What we now know is that, if you lose this finger, your visual cortex doesn't start responding to stimulation, taking over. But we do see that there is evidence now that the auditory cortex is getting inputs from the somatosensory cortex, from the visual cortex; that the boundaries between the senses are not as cleanly divided as we once thought.

There are probably reasons for that. We're always trying to integrate information across senses and information is getting integrated across different systems, so you want some feed-forward and feedback information crossing over.

HB: And you want some redundancy.

GH: Yes, you want some redundancy. That could be one of the mechanisms of plasticity. You've got these—not quite latent, but, let's say—undercurrent of connections, so that if the normal inputs go away, you've got other systems that can generate information being sent into this area. That could be functional or not. It could wire up to some system that actually leads to adaptive behaviour, or it might get used and actually interfere with it.

HB: So if that's right, then another question is, *How broad is this?* As you were saying just now, it's probably not the visual cortex that somehow links to your pinky, but I'm wondering, *How do you impose boundaries—how broad can it be?*

GH: Yes. Back in the 1990s, people were very interested in plasticity in the neocortex and how flexible these systems seemed to be.

For example, V.S. Ramachandran at UCSD demonstrated really interesting things. People who were amputees felt their limb on their face. You could actually touch their cheek and they would feel stimulation in their missing finger. What he found was that in some people a map of a hand was on the face. That made sense because things overlapped and those areas are near each other.

This was taken as an example of the dramatic plasticity of the cortex, that things can take over function. I always wondered why the cortex persisted in perceiving something that isn't there anymore. *What is it that's making it want to perceive that still, that you would still get it?* So I was always more interested in the constraints on plasticity. *What stops it from just being a Wild West?*

HB: And also why there? Why on the cheek? Not just why not the hand, but why that particular place as opposed to somewhere else?

GH: Right. So there are some constraints on it. That's interesting. I don't know that we know the answer to that. I certainly don't, maybe someone else does.

HB: People are still working on it, though, right? This wasn't solved in the 1990s and I missed it entirely?

GH: No: there's lots of plasticity work still going on.

Questions for Discussion:

1. Why is it so clear to both Greg and Howard that redundancy in brain processing systems is advantageous? Might that not be viewed as inefficient?

2. How might a deeper understanding of neuroplasticity be harnessed for future medical treatments?

X. On the Front Burner

Lots to investigate

HB: One last issue before we conclude, if I may, I'd like to turn to your current research and what you're working on now. Let me ask a very specific question that I tend to bombard people with at the end of these conversations: if I were an omniscient being and could give you the answer to any research question you might have, what would you ask me? What are the things keeping you up at night?

GH: What are the things keeping me up at night? I work in language and speech, and I'm basically trying to map out the circuits involved in sensory motor control. That's one major focus of my work. Another focus is trying to figure out how the auditory system works and is organized at a fairly basic level.

There are a lot of people working on speech who are interested in finding areas that are involved in phonological processing and things like that, and there's a lot of work in hearing generally. People are interested in cochlear dynamics and all sorts of specific, low-level things.

How those things actually come together is something that's very interesting to me. We've been doing some work trying to map out the auditory cortex, what the maps look like. We think we've identified another dimension of the auditory cortex that's not just tonotopy: it's basically a time dimension that the auditory cortex codes in the maps. We've been working on that and trying to think about how that relates to our ability to perceive speech sounds and frequency, the frequency-time relation.

That's one thing that I'm interested in. There's a lot of work, a lot of excitement in neuroscience, regarding neural oscillation: the tendency for brain systems to oscillate and how that might be playing a role in cognition or perception.

HB: I don't know what that means. What are the neural systems that are oscillating?

GH: If you record from individual neurons—let's just take EEG as the obvious example: just stick an electrode on your head and record the brainwaves. They're not random. They tend to oscillate at particular frequencies.

The question is, *Why are they doing that? Is it helpful in computation?* There's a lot of evidence that's actually part of the way the brain either codes information or primes the system for processing information at the relevant time points, as we're processing information over time.

There's a lot of interest in that, which is perhaps connected to the time maps we've identified in the auditory cortex. Or maybe not. We're trying to work out some of those details.

So those are some of the questions that I'm worried about. I'm trying to work out how networks might be wired up to support our ability to perceive and produce speech sounds, which is a ridiculously complex task and can be easily disrupted with brain damage and leave people devastated without language. It would be nice to work out those circuits; then perhaps we can come up with a device, a neural prosthesis, for rewiring brains.

HB: When you're looking at these circuits, are you looking at them being localized in particular areas? I mean, there are the obvious areas that seem to be predominantly associated with speech and so forth. Are they more localized in those areas, or are they spread out fairly widely throughout the brain?

GH: Well, they're distributed networks that have nodes in them, typically. For the sensory network in speech we think we've identified the relevant network, at least in broad strokes.

We can point to those areas, and the game is trying to figure out what those different networks are doing: how the system operates as a whole together with trying to calculate what it's actually doing.

I'm spending a lot of time working on trying to integrate motor control with all of this. There's a lot of work on the engineering of how to control and optimize a robotic arm and how the brain might be doing that.

Then there are people who are studying these processes from a linguistic perspective. I see this as an opportunity to put those pieces together and try to come up with an integrated picture of how the brain might be doing this for speech. We're making some progress, I think.

HB: Very interesting. One more question. Recently I talked to Diana Deutsch about her work in auditory illusions (see the Ideas Roadshow conversation *Believing Your Ears: Examining Auditory Illusions*), and in that conversation we discussed how auditory illusions might be able to shine a light, as it were, on the different auditory processing systems in the brain.

There's this notion that there may be different auditory systems, —analogous to the different visual systems—and that these auditory illusions might be able to somehow evaluate and measure these different systems.

Is that something that would be interesting to you? Are others involved in that sort of thing? Is that a tool that people could or should be using in your view?

GH: Well, illusions have been used in visual science for a long time to help try to figure out how this system is organized, and I know Diana Deutsch has been very active in uncovering auditory illusions.

They haven't been utilized as much in auditory work to the best of my knowledge. But I don't see any reason why they couldn't be.

In fact, some of the principles that Diana's work suggested decades ago are principles that are being developed now, even in my own work. Years ago she talked about the idea that there were two auditory systems, organized functionally differently, and one of the big things that I've been promoting over the last decade is the idea of dorsal sensory motor stream that's coming out of the auditory system versus a ventral stream that has different functions.

This parallels the visual system and probably is a general principle of how the brain works with respect to processing sensory information.

I don't see any reason why that sort of information couldn't be utilized and put to good use in auditory work.

HB: Anything else? Anything we missed? Anything you'd like to add?

GH: No, I think we covered just about all of it.

HB: Great. Thanks a lot, Greg. That was a lot of fun.

GH: Yes, that was a lot of fun. Thank you.

Questions for Discussion:

1. In general, to what extent do you think that a better understanding of one brain system will shed light on another? Might it one day be appropriate not to look at any one "brain system" at all?

2. What sorts of experiments would you be most interested in doing if you were in Greg's shoes?

Continuing the Conversation

Readers are encouraged to read Greg's book, *The Myth of Mirror Neurons: The Real Neuroscience of Communication and Cognition*, which goes into considerable additional detail about many of the issues discussed here.

Exploring Autism

A conversation with Uta Frith

Introduction
The Autistic Condition

Autism, it seems, is all around us. Once thought to only affect a tiny minority of 0.04% of the population, modern researchers are now of the view that it is more than 25 times more prevalent than we had once imagined, with current figures estimating that more than 1% of us suffer from autism-type disorders. So what is going on? Are we in the throes of an "autism epidemic"?

Uta Frith of UCL's Institute of Cognitive Neuroscience and one of the world's leading experts on autism, says no. The vastly increased number of autism diagnoses is simply a reflection of our growing awareness of a condition whose breadth has led modern researchers to begin referring to an autism spectrum rather than one specific affliction. Many people who are now considered autistic would have remained undiagnosed had they been born in an earlier time.

> *"People often find the fact that we didn't know about autism before very strange. They say: 'Well, suddenly we hear all about autism; it didn't use to be around'. But the answer is quite simply that people had no way of talking about these particular individuals, these particular children. Of course, the parents were aware of this and they had to deal with this forever. It isn't a new phenomenon: it's just newly addressed and newly labelled."*

So no epidemic, then. But still: what are we really talking about? What is autism, anyway?

This seemingly obvious first step, Uta carefully stresses, turns out to be a surprisingly hard question to comprehensively answer

"You might say,: 'Hey, after all this time, you should come up with a definition: you should really know what it is', but people are still arguing about it. But I will give you what I think is the core of what autism is, the kind of essence of autism.

I believe it is a neurologically-caused entity that I would describe as lacking the otherwise innate ability to attribute an inner life to other people and to oneself: mental states, feelings, ideas, knowledge and so on."

In fact, Uta and her colleagues actually coined a new word, *mentalize*, to refer to this ability based on a series of groundbreaking experiments on autistic children in the 1980s.

*"**Mentalizing** is a completely made-up word, and we had to make up a word because people hadn't been talking about this ability before; this ability to attribute mental states to others, now sometimes called 'theory of mind'."*

Perhaps the best way to develop a deep appreciation of what mentalizing means is to return to those experiments that gave rise to the concept in the first place, the most famous of which is the so-called Sally-Anne Test, where children are presented with specifically constructed social situations acted out by two dolls, Sally and Anne.

"Sally has this marble and she puts the marble into her basket and now she wants to go out and play, so she leaves the scene and goes completely away. Meanwhile, naughty Anne goes to the basket, takes out that marble and puts it into her own box.

"Now it's time for Sally to come back. She comes back and she wants to play with her marble.

"Now we ask the child, who has been watching this scene unfold: where will Sally look for her marble?

*"The ordinary child would say that Sally should naturally look in her basket, because she has no way of knowing that Anne has taken the marble away. Sally has a **false belief** that lets you predict what she*

will do. Sally will look there and will not find the marble; all the while the child knows where the marble really is.

"But the majority of the autistic children, about three quarters of them, gave the wrong answer. They said, 'Sally will look here in Anne's box'.

*"In other words, in a situation which might well occur in real life, they couldn't make the right prediction of where a person will look, what a person will do. They would get it **wrong**.*

*"Their predictions for the behaviour of others would simply be in terms of what **they** know, what it is in **their** reality. And that is exactly what this special innate mechanism allows us to overcome."*

So that's it then, one might be tempted to conclude: what distinguishes us from autistic people is our ability to mentalize, to look at things from someone else's viewpoint.

Not so fast, says Professor Frith. There are, she believes, two quite different ways of mentalizing. Attributing mental states to others is sometimes done in a very conscious, deliberate way. After all, that is exactly what successful advertisers do as they methodically go about trying to find the most effective way to "get into our heads". And it turns out that some autistic people—particularly those with high intelligence—can do this as well. But from a neurophysiological level, this conscious, rational way of mentalizing is not the same thing as its intuitive, spontaneous, innate mentalizing counterpart.

Indeed, brain scans reveal that, while all mentalizing activities have a characteristic brain signature, those advanced autistic patients who are engaging in a more conscious, effortful type of mentalizing don't seem to display the same neural signature as that of those who are mentalizing unconsciously. It is as if the connectivity between different areas of the brain is somehow weaker.

Intriguingly too, autistic children don't always underperform in tests with their non-autistic counterparts. In particular, autistic children consistently outperform others when it comes to puzzles geared towards finding hidden shapes, or figures, in an overall picture.

These results led Uta to develop her theory of *Weak Central Coherence* (WCC), the notion that the autistic mind naturally focuses on the details rather than the whole. This peculiarity can be readily grasped in a visual setting, like trying to locate hidden shapes in a puzzle, but can also be generalized to more abstract arenas, such as language, where autism is typically associated with an undue emphasis on the literal and a lack of understanding of a broader overall context.

Weak Central Coherence, Uta is quick to point out, is only a hypothesis and is far from universally accepted throughout the scientific community. But one of the things that particularly intrigues me about the theory is that it has helped to move the autism goalposts away from simple declarations of the lack of mentalizing capacities to a more subtle analysis of the spectrum of human types.

As is generally appreciated, the tendency to focus intently on specific details is often linked with extreme accomplishments in music, art, mathematics and many other fields of human endeavour. Indeed, Hans Asperger, one of the founders of autism research in the 1940s, famously mused that autistic intelligence represents an extreme form of intelligence, while the popular consciousness has long been captivated by the notion of *Rain Man* and other, so-called "idiots savants".

More generally, some psychological researchers speculate that the tendency towards detail or Gestalt thinking is nothing more than a basic human characteristic: that each of us naturally finds ourselves at some point on the continuum between the two extremes of "detail obsessiveness" and "vague generalities".

Clearly there is much more to autism than simply a statistical grouping of those who find themselves at one end of some mental categorization scheme, but the important thing to bear in mind is that further research might do much more than give us a clearer understanding of the fundamental nature of this mysterious condition.

It could well give us a clearer understanding about ourselves.

The Conversation

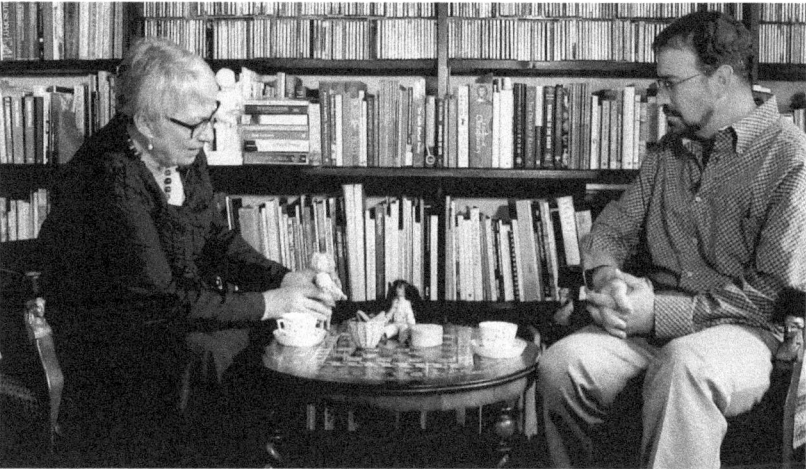

I. Assessing the Landscape

An autism epidemic?

HB: It's a real pleasure for me to have a chance to talk to you in your lovely home about autism, a subject that you've devoted a large proportion of your research career to.

UF: Well, I'm naturally very pleased that you take such an interest in autism. While many people are talking now about autism, there is usually some sort of political agenda associated with it and the actual science is perhaps less well known.

HB: We were speaking earlier before we started filming about the cultural difference, as it were, between science and what often gets communicated to the general public.

In science, of course, it's perfectly acceptable to admit that one doesn't know something and highlight the current outstanding mysteries, but in the media or general public consciousness, often admitting one's ignorance is often strongly frowned upon as a sign of incompetence.

UF: Yes. The world of research is very, very different in these matters, as you say.

I can talk about my own research, which goes back nearly 50 years now, really quite a long time. And very often I say to myself: *"Well, I've been at this problem for so long, I've been trying to find reasons why we find all these phenomena in autism and I **still** don't know, even now I **still** don't know."*

Even now, when I see a new person with autism I find something surprising. Of course this is also the thing that has made me highly curious and passionate about trying to find out a little bit more about it.

If I had known in the late 60s, when I started to be interested in the topic, that even after all this time it would still be such a mystery—or enigma, as we sometimes call it—I would not have believed it. I would have thought that, surely, we will first of all find the causes in biology in the brain and in the genes. And we will also find some kind of treatment, some best possible way forward, and we will have a good theory about the mind in autism: how it works.

But it is not as simple as that, because when you start talking about phenomena in autism and the special mysteries there, you're really talking about mysteries of the human mind, and that is such a big topic that a period of 50 years is absolutely nothing. When you think about how long it took us to understand the cosmos—and even that is an ongoing project—

HB: Even balls falling. I mean, even basic mechanics took a very long time to fully understand.

UF: Yes. And as far as our study of the mind is concerned, we've only *just* started; we've only just begun. I think many people don't quite appreciate how recent, for example, psychiatry is.

Even scientifically-based medicine is quite recent: we haven't had that for more than about 400 years or so, but psychiatry—scientific attempts to treat disorders of the mind, of the brain—is barely a hundred years old.

That's also one of the reasons why we didn't know about autism before. People often find that very strange. They say: "*Well, suddenly we hear all about autism; it didn't use to be around*". But the answer is quite simply that people had *no way of talking* about these particular individuals, these particular children. Of course, the parents were aware of this and they had to deal with this forever. It isn't a new phenomenon: it's just newly addressed and newly labelled.

HB: That's interesting, because when *I* started delving deeper into the subject of autism—which was a matter of weeks ago rather than a matter of decades ago—my reaction was very much as you described. All of a sudden it seemed to me that everybody is talking about this— autism, Asperger syndrome, and so forth—it seems to be all around us.

UF: Yes.

HB: And if you don't know anything about these things, you're hearing these words being thrown around all over the place and there's this sense of almost scaremongering with people saying: "*We're in the midst of an autism epidemic!*"

UF: Right. Suddenly it's there and it's increasing rapidly: *I know people who have an autistic child. Could it happen to me? Could it happen to my family?*

HB: Exactly.

UF: Well, first of all, I think that in the past there was a lot of suppression of mental illness in general. It was very, very heavily stigmatized—it was a very big problem of dealing with an otherwise healthy child who had real problems with language, with learning, with social interaction. People didn't know what to do or what to think about that.

In fact there were, in pre-scientific days, stories of possession, stories of "the changeling child". People could not easily cope with this kind of problem; and at the time when I started my PhD research in the 1960s, there were very big institutions for mentally-handicapped children and mentally-handicapped adults. They were put out of sight, out of mind: around the periphery of London there were some of these huge institutions—asylums—where a large number of children were placed whom I believe were autistic.

When we first started our research, we thought autism concerned a particular subgroup, a possibly tiny group out of this huge bulk of what was called "mental retardation", and that we might be able to develop some angle on it to find some understanding of what in the brain went wrong.

A large proportion of this mentally-retarded population had definite brain pathology that you could see under the microscope after they died. But there are also cases—and autism is a particular example—where you couldn't see anything with the naked eye: the brain seemed perfectly fine.

In order to get a deeper understanding of what people thought, it's important to appreciate that there was still this idea of something we call 'dualism': the belief that there is a clear distinction between "*the body*" as represented by "*the brain*" and "*the mind*".

Many believed that you could have mental disorders that have nothing to do with your body and your brain, mental disorders that had mental causes, psychological causes which would have nothing to do with any kind of biological or neurological involvement—

HB: Just mind stuff.

UF: Right: just mind stuff.

And the main theory that was quite dominant for a while, and is still fighting to be heard, is this idea that it's all to do with a trauma that a child experiences, perhaps in not being bonded with the mother properly, possibly rejected by the mother.

The idea wasn't that this was a necessarily conscious act on the mother's part, but rather some kind of deep psychoanalytic process that made the mother reject the child.

And so psychoanalysts concluded that they could cure autism by treating the mother and the child; they thought there was absolutely nothing wrong with that person, neurologically speaking.

That was real, plain dualism which we now completely reject, because we now believe that there *is* a connection between the mind and the brain.

HB: Well, not everyone, I should interject, as you well know: in 2011 the filmmaker Sophie Robert released a documentary (*The Wall*) describing how many people in France still treat autism according to the way you described: from a psychoanalytical perspective as opposed to a neurobiological one.

UF: Yes, unfortunately this is still going on, even though there is absolutely no scientific evidence for it; and that, I think, is quite scandalous. I mean, it is really quackery, there is just no other word for it.

There are people who really believe, and parents who really believe, that maybe by some kind of power of the talking cure you could somehow suddenly have some kind of normal person emerging—well, maybe not suddenly, but at least gradually.

They reject the idea that there is a neurological basis that gives certain limitations on what you can do and not do, and what you should accept as given and what you have to work with, rather than wishing to change the autistic person somehow from autistic into something else.

HB: Right. But let me now return to my level of confusion that I referred to earlier: I'm hearing all this talk about autism, but I don't really know what it is.

UF: Right.

HB: So let me try to briefly summarize your views based upon what I've been reading and watching and you can tell me if I've got it right or wrong.

UF: OK.

HB: My understanding is that you believe that there is no "autism epidemic" at all, and there are two distinct reasons why it appears to us that autism is much more prevalent today than it was in the past.

First, there has been a relabelling of psychological cases, so that those who were previously regarded as "mentally retarded" or something else are now regarded as autistic.

And secondly, there are many more subtle and less obvious aspects of what constitutes autism that in the past wouldn't have been diagnosed or perhaps even noticed.

UF: You got that absolutely right.

There has been a widening of what can be called autism into a whole spectrum as it's called—sometimes people say it's actually *autisms* in plural. Of those who were previously grouped into the category of being "mentally handicapped" or "intellectually disabled", many can now be given the label "autism" on the grounds of some different specific clinical criteria.

But at the same time, we go to the opposite extreme, and we look at people who are highly intelligent, often very eccentric (those we have long known about in novels and from family histories), and suddenly these people are *also* called "autistic" because there are certain features in their behaviour.

For example, a very obsessive interest in a particular topic, a very narrow and rigid style of life and a social awkwardness, and a lack of interest in social communication, that all seem to make us ask: *"Well, isn't that just a version of what can be described as the essence of autism that applies to people in this whole spectrum?"*

Now, having made it so wide, of course, you can see that more and more cases will be labelled like that. So this accounts for the steep increase that we suddenly get, just because people are now given this label that they would never have been given before.

Once this happened, it was almost like an avalanche, because suddenly people—psychiatrists for example—thought: *Yes, we have these patients that we've never quite been able to classify, they fit into* ***that*** *category.*

And there were parents who said: "*Well, my son is very strange and he just doesn't have friends, and all he is interested in is trains*", and now there was a sense that this was a condition that could actually been given a label so that the child would finally be able to get special consideration and special help.

So there has naturally been much motivation for pushing for more diagnoses and that's why we have an increasing number of cases. Of course, there is a limit, there is a ceiling that will be reached beyond which there won't be any more cases.

Questions for Discussion:

1. Do you believe there is a difference between "the brain" and "the mind"? Is this view reinforced by contemporary societal, cultural and religious views?

2. How can we be certain that the absolute number of autism cases isn't increasing if we have no clear baseline of how many there were in the past?

II. Searching for a Definition

Innate vs. conscious understanding

HB: I'd like to ask you more about that, because from my layman's perspective I might say, "*OK, I understand that the definitions have evolved, more cases are been taken into consideration, there's a broader understanding of this phenomenon and so forth, but where is the limit? Perhaps I could simply let matters evolve indefinitely, so that one day everybody in the world might be considered a little bit or a lot autistic?*"

After all, if we're to be proper scientists, we have to have some reasonably clearer definition, or cut-off, of what this condition actually is and what it means to have it.

UF: I agree.

HB: So when I ask you, as an expert in autism research: what *is* it; what is autism, exactly? How would you respond?

UF: It is not an easy question.

HB: Sure. But it's not my job to ask easy questions.

UF: You might say,: "*Hey, after all this time, you should come up with a definition: you should really know what it is*", but people are *still* arguing about it.

But I'll give you what I think— and many others will agree—is the *core* of what autism is, the kind of essence of autism.

I believe it is a neurologically caused entity: I believe there is, ultimately, a genetic (plus potentially environmental) cause well before birth—we're not talking about environmental causes due to maternal rejection or anything like that.

And I would characterize this entity as lacking the otherwise innate ability—and that's quite a big claim which is still controversial—to attribute an inner life to other people and to oneself: mental states, feelings, ideas, knowledge and so on.

Now this innate ability is not something necessarily uniquely human. This is something that has been observed in a variety of other species.

Take crows. These birds seem to be able to take into account whether another bird observes them while they are hiding some food; and after the other bird has left, they will go and put that food somewhere else so that it can't be stolen.

This is what I mean by that innate ability to attribute, in this case knowledge of what's happening to another agent of your own species. And most human infants can do that too.

I believe that autistic infants are *not* born with this ability, and therefore it puts development onto quite a different track.

So the way, for example, that we normally learn language is also by attributing knowledge to another person or having some joint interest in understanding, which is all done totally unconsciously.

Now this ability has major repercussions, because it drives all our interest in communicating our inner thoughts because we know we have different thoughts in our heads.

I can't assume that you think the same as I do. You have a different field of view: for example, you see these dolls on the table between us from the back while I see them from the front. I can make these allowances for the differences between your point of view and my point of view without thinking about it. This is just sort of "built in".

HB: It is innate.

UF: Yes. And I think that this is *not* innate and "built into" the autistic brain.

But that's not all: that's the underlying theory, the idea, that can explain a particular, very specific inability to communicate, together with a style of social interaction that is typically associated with autism. But it is important to emphasize here that it's *not* true that people with autism are asocial, antisocial, socially disinterested, not socially aware: all of this is just *not true*.

There are some very specific things that they find very difficult to do in social interactions that turn out to be terribly important, so important that they are done at this unconscious level.

Because of its importance, evolution has not left this to chance and left us to learn about it over a period of years in some kind of trial and error way—no, most of us can do it right away. It's very subtle but it's also very pervasive: we can immediately see that other agents have motives to do certain things: intentions, beliefs and desires just like we have intentions, beliefs and desires.

Now what's interesting about humans—and this is perhaps unique to humans—is that they can also *reflect upon* this ability; they can think about it. Just like how I'm talking about it now, we can discuss in a perfectly rational way how your point of view is different from my point of view: I can imagine what your view is, and what my view is, all in a very conscious way.

So we can do this, but it turns out that it's *not the same thing* as this intuitive, spontaneous, automatic, innate ability to attribute mental states to other people. And very interestingly, this conscious way of talking about mental states is open to be learned—slowly and effortfully—to people with autism.

I think I should explain this a little bit more because it may seem a bit too mysterious. This is a relatively new development of these ideas, making a distinction between the implicit unconscious way of attributing mental states and the conscious way of doing so. The important thing to emphasize is that the conscious way is possible to acquire even if you are autistic, even if you don't have that intuitive sense.

HB: But presumably not all people with autism can do this, not all of them can consciously construct this sense of looking at things from another point of view.

UF: They have to have a certain degree of cognitive ability. This is where those on the very clever end will shine: they will use all their intelligence, their resources, their ability for making inferences, for understanding what goes on in these sorts of situations. They will learn it and they can become absolutely perfect at it.

HB: Absolutely perfect? That was my next question: since it's learned behaviour, will they be able to do it in a way where nobody could actually tell that they have autism? In other words, would they be *absolutely perfect* or is it more the case that they would be able to simulate it to a high degree?

UF: They would be able to do it perfectly if it was done in writing. If you did it by email, for example. It is important to have enough time to think things through appropriately. It is still quite possible in a conversation given sufficient time to respond and consider because many of these situations have already been rehearsed in various tests. They can do those tests perfectly because they've studied them and read about them. So in a sense they've lost their potential to be sensitive in a diagnostic sense.

It is wonderfully positive and encouraging that this can be learned behaviour, but I insist that it's *not the same thing*.

When we also do this consciously—give an answer that's reflective—that takes a little bit of time and this is perhaps quite separate and quite divorced from our sort of intuitive way of attributing mental states that we probably never give up entirely. We use, I think, both these levels at the same time.

But if you are autistic, you just have that very effortful, conscious level that engages your intellectual abilities quite a lot, while if you also had that intuitive level you might well be able to do other things and think other thoughts at the same time. So it's a much less effortful way of doing these things and stands us in quite good stead.

Like all innate things, it can sometimes be for the good, and sometimes be for the bad. And these conscious actions too can sometimes be for the bad, sometimes for the good.

Take the example of Machiavelli, who wrote this famous book giving advice to the Prince of how best to get ahead in a political climate, how to be an effective ruler and how to see through other people. Today we use the word "Machiavellian" as a way of manipulating others. Well, advertising people do that all very, very consciously. They know what works. So this is all to do with this conscious part of attributing mental states and we *do* use it. And we sometimes have quite a struggle, I think, to turn off the power of advertising: to say to ourselves: "*I have to resist this because this is just pure manipulation*".

HB: "*They're getting into my head*".

UF: Yes. But if you can *only* connect on this totally intuitive level, then it's very difficult to resist anything, then you're caught. So the real danger is that one person is consciously manipulating, while the other person is being purely intuitive and is completely unaware of what is happening.

Questions for Discussion:

1. How might this "innate ability" to attribute an inner life to others be linked to "social intelligence"?

2. Might there be a way of objectively distinguishing between the "innate" and "conscious" way of attributing an inner life to others by, say, using brain-imaging technology?

III. A Stunning Result

Learning from dolls

HB: This idea that you've called "theory of mind" and "mentalizing"—this notion of being able to understand other people's perspectives, their desires, their intentions and so forth that autistic people do not innately have—

UF: Well, I'd like to emphasize that it's still a theory.

HB: OK. It's worth highlighting that everything I say should really be prefaced with *"That you believe".*

UF: Yes. I believe that. Not everybody believes it, but it seems to be more accepted than not after about 30 years of pretty severe testing trying to demolish it.

HB: Right. So that's where I'm going. I'm summarizing the claim—and it *is* a claim—that a key distinguishing feature between autistic people and those who are not autistic is that those who are autistic do not have the ability to be able to *mentalize*, to be able to ascribe beliefs and intentions to other people—

UF: In an intuitive fashion.

HB: Right: in an intuitive, innate fashion. Although, as you've just been emphasizing, some *are* able to compensate by doing this consciously.

UF: Yes, some can.

HB: OK. But putting that aside for the moment, autistic people lack this innate ability.

UF: Which has a neurological basis. It's some kind of system in the brain that probably evolved relatively late, as far as we can tell, because it's likely not pervasive in all animal species.

So here we are: this little bit of brain system is not working as it should in the autistic brain.

HB: So this is the claim. But what I think is particularly important to stress here is that this is a claim that has been supported experimentally, both in terms of rigorous experimental psychological tests of behaviour—which I would like you to explain in more detail shortly—and also in terms of neurological examinations involving brain-imaging technology.

UF: Yes. So, "mentalizing" is a completely made-up word: we had to make up a word because people hadn't been talking about this ability before; this ability to attribute mental states to others, sometimes called "theory of mind".

There is a specific test with dolls which, I think, makes this all more concrete.

This is the scenario: we have these two dolls who perform a little act in front of some four-year-old children. The first experiment was done in 1983 or 1984 by Simon Baron-Cohen for his PhD thesis.

Anyway, you don't have to use dolls of course, you can use real people, you can use all sorts of things. But let's get back to the test: there is one doll called Sally and another called Anne. Sally has a basket and Anne has a box.

Sally has this marble and she puts it into her basket. Now she wants to go out and play, so she leaves the scene and goes completely away. Meanwhile, naughty Anne goes to the basket, takes out that marble and puts it into her own box.

Now it's time for Sally to come back. She comes back and she wants to play with her marble. Now we ask the child, who's been watching the entire scene unfold, *"Where will Sally look for her marble?"*

The ordinary child would say that Sally should look in her basket, because she has *no way of knowing* that Anne has taken the marble away. Sally has a false belief—that's why it's often called a "false belief test"—and that false belief lets you predict what she will do. It makes the right prediction: Sally will look there and will not find the marble; all the while the child knows where the marble really is.

And we ask the child that explicitly just to confirm that and ensure that there is no misunderstanding. We ask, *"Where was the marble, really?"* and the child will reply, *"It's in Anne's box."*

HB: So the normal child will understand that Sally would believe, with complete justification, that the marble would still be in her basket?

UF: That's right, yes.

HB: So once again, just to be very explicit, the normal child is, as it were, "getting into the head" of Sally and looking at things from Sally's perspective.

UF: Yes. Now this experiment was actually devised by two extremely clever psychologists, Josef Perner and Heinz Wimmer in Austria. They used it with normal children to study development.

They said: *"Most five-year olds get this, most three-year olds are just completely at odds with it, and then of course older children wouldn't want to play such a childish game."*

We were so happy to have that paradigm when Simon Baron-Cohen started his thesis under the supervision of myself and Alan Leslie. We thought that this experiment should be done with autistic children, although I predicted they would be able to do it, actually.

HB: Really? So you were quite surprised by the results?

UF: I was very, very surprised. These were quite clever children: they had good language, they had good memory.

But what, in fact, Simon found in his experiments was that the majority of the autistic children, about three quarters of them, gave the wrong answer. They said, *"Sally will look here in Anne's box."*

And of course you can ask different variations of the question like, *"Where does Sally think the marble is?"* but very often when this type of experiment was repeated, the autistic children didn't seem to take the belief of another agent into account; instead they acted according to reality.

The real state of affairs was: *here is the marble in the box, not in the basket.* So in other words, in a situation which might well occur in real life, they couldn't make the right prediction of where a person will look, what a person will do. They would get it *wrong.*

Their predictions for the behaviour of others would simply be in terms of what they know, what it is in their reality. And that is exactly what this special innate mechanism allows us to overcome.

So beliefs are more important than reality in these situations. Alan Leslie always used this example: *Why does John go out with an umbrella? It's not because it's raining, but rather because he* **believes** *it will rain.*

That's why he takes the umbrella, *that's* how you can predict his actions. In fact, you can predict he'll take an umbrella if you know he doesn't want to get wet, so this is also a reflection of his desires. You can attribute desires, just like beliefs, to other people; and this is how you go about the social world.

This was the starting point for "theory of mind", and how important we believed that it was to understand autism. It was also the starting point of us asking: *"What on earth enables young children— and adults too, of course—to think that way?"*

And the really daring hypothesis was that there is a special brain mechanism for it. Most people thought this was crazy. Most people thought along the lines of, *Everything is conscious inference: hundreds of things must be in place before this can be done. You need to be at age four to put 2 and 2 together and you do it with all of your brain:*

you use your language, your memory, and then you add it all together and you solve this problem.

Now after all these decades of research I think most people have now agreed that: "*No, you don't have to do this in a conscious way. If you are not autistic, you can do this in a sort of shortcut way without thinking about it consciously.*"

And others have shown that very young babies, aged seven months or so, act in a way, just by looking, where they appear to anticipate actions on the basis of somebody's belief ,rather than, say, on the basis of actions.

HB: That's fascinating. Even though they can't yet speak, we can still tell just by their eye movements and their facial expressions—

UF: Yes. This is a different kind of experimentation that was done outside the field of autism to find out how these things develop in ordinary cognitive development.

What we tried to study directly was the neurological underpinning of this ability to mentalize; a pretty daring thing to do, pretty high risk.

HB: High risk perhaps, but it seems to me that this is the way science is done.

And you had a groundbreaking result: you had experimental evidence, clear statistical evidence, to support the distinction between the actions of autistic and non-autistic children.

You were in a position to say: "*Here's a revealing experiment that we can perform that shows a clear behavioural difference.*"

Different people might interpret the results in different ways—you're constructing this idea of the "theory of mind" or "mentalizing" to shed light on things—but clearly there is *something* very noteworthy going on. That must have been extremely exciting to recognize.

UF: It was extremely exciting. And it was then possible to further test the idea because we suddenly had the brain scanners. People were asked to think about a scenario like this Sally-Anne experiment and then we could see what the brain does.

Questions for Discussion:

1. What does Uta mean by "a special brain mechanism" and why do you think that she feels that was "a really daring hypothesis"? How, if at all, do you think the notion of dualism between the mind and the brain is relevant to this issue?

2. To what extent can the phrase, "Beliefs are more important than reality in these situations" be applied to a wealth of models in economics, politics and other areas of the social sciences? What, if anything, might this imply about the importance of "theory of mind" more generally?

IV. Looking Inside

Brain-imaging technology and its impact

HB: So what happens?

UF: Well, before I tell you about the results, let me first tell you about how it works, which relies upon this key concept of "subtraction". You can't see anything if you just look at the brain: the brain is just terribly active. So that's not the way to use the technique. The technique is used by asking people to think about something that's incredibly similar but doesn't involve mentalizing so that you can compare the two results and identify the mentalizing part.

HB: So how would that work, exactly?

UF: In our first experiment using brain scanners we used little stories that people read. One story would be, for example, the Sally-Anne story or something like that. It was actually done with completely healthy adults—they just read this little story and then we asked them a question: *Why did Sally look in her basket?*

They're thinking silently; and, of course, their brain is active all over the place. Then we had little stories that concerned factual, mechanical things: John goes to the store to buy some light bulbs, but he only has enough money to buy a certain number, or something like that.

So then what we had to do was subtract the brain activity of one kind of thinking about one kind of story, from that of another kind of thinking about a different type of story, and see what we had left and what the difference was.

HB: So you have a sort of mask that lets you distinguish between the mentalizing brain and the non-mentalizing brain.

UF: Exactly. And even in that very first study, which was very tentative, we actually found a particular network involving the frontal, temporal and parietal lobes of the brain—different locations that were nonetheless interconnected. That seemed to be the one thing that was active over and above what's active for working out the solution to a particular problem as presented in a normal, straightforward little story.

After this, lots of other materials have been used—pictures, cartoon stories, moving triangles—that always involve a subtraction, a comparison, of one task requiring mentalizing with another similar task that does not requiring mentalizing.

And that's how we can fathom that there is something extra to this process of mentalizing.

HB: That's a fantastic result.

UF: It is very exciting; but remember it's not as exciting as it could be because in order to get this result we had to sum up the average of the brain activity from a whole lot of people. We can't do this for each individual person. Furthermore, we can't do it for a particular story either. We have to summarize it over twelve stories of one kind and then twelve stories of another kind. There is a lot of noise there.

The instruments are just not good enough to do this in a way where you could say, "*Look at my brain. Am I now mentalizing or not?*" We're not there yet. The instruments are not microscopic enough. If I do this with you a hundred times—and then you might get bored and not actually think the way I want you to think—and then I compared this with you thinking a hundred times about other types of stories, and then I subtracted them, maybe I could see something.

HB: But that's very suggestive nonetheless.

I do actually want to talk a little bit about the brain scan technology in itself and how it works, because this is something that I was certainly not aware of, and it's fascinating in its own right.

But first I think it's important to emphasize the central result: that however limited we are by the current level of technology, there seems to be a strong statistical correlation that leads us to conclude that when people are mentalizing they are using a different aspect of their brain, different areas of their brain, than when they are not.

UF: That's exactly so. This system has been verified again and again. It is there when you think about yourself, when you do all sorts of similar mentalizing tasks and compare these to other contrasting, non-mentalizing activities. But of course we also looked at autistic people doing the same thing.

Once again the autistic people we worked with are these very, very clever people who can think consciously about these sorts of things as we said earlier. Of course they got the right answers—as I said earlier, if they have enough time, they will definitely get the right answers to these sorts of questions—but the corresponding activity in the brain—again, over a whole group of people, over a whole lot of stories—was less. It was reduced. It's a little bit puzzling because the results seem to be telling us that they have the same network but it's not working as efficiently somehow.

People have shown this again and again: it's not quite the same activation pattern. The best possible guess at the moment—again, backed by evidence—is that the connectivity between the different areas is very weak in the case of autism. So it seems that, in the case of autism, the system is somehow just not properly connected together.

HB: So, just to summarize again: you have similar types of activation in the brain for autistic people who are doing these mentalizing experiments?

UF: Yes.

HB: But not quite to the same extent somehow. There seem to be differences related to how the connectivity between the different regions across the network is working.

UF: That's right.

HB: And of course you know, or at least are strongly convinced, from doing your Sally-Anne experiments and other experiments, that there is a deep difference in this mentalizing ability between those who are autistic and those who are not.

UF: Yes.

HB: And now, in addition to experimental psychological evidence, you have some neurophysiological evidence that reinforces your view that there is, statistically speaking at least, a genuine difference there.

UF: Yes, absolutely. I totally believe in that; and in fact I would make a bet that, with better instruments, we will get a much clearer view of the situation: we shall really see what's going on.

One of the things that has not yet been done is to conduct a study with truly intuitive mentalizing. Most of the studies that have been done actually allow this explicit, conscious mentalizing to happen, because they're slow, they present the material in a sort of conscious way, so the autistic people who are in the scanner can actually do a lot by way of compensation.

We have no way of knowing yet how their brains would respond to a truly implicit, quick, intuitive task. I think this is where we should find the biggest difference.

HB: We're still quite limited by the technology.

UF: Yes.

HB: One of the things that is also probably worth explicitly highlighting at this point is what these brain scans are actually doing.

My naive view, when I first heard about brain scans, is that there is now a way to get some sort of snapshot of the neurological activity in the brain and see which regions, perhaps even which individual neurons, are firing—

UF: Like an X-ray: being able to examine if the bone structure is right or wrong.

HB: Exactly.

UF: Well, that's what we want these brain imaging methods to be like in the future. But we're not there yet. There is a huge gap between directly recording the activities of neurons and our present technology: right now it's all about blood flow.

HB: Right; that's what I was completely ignorant of. Not too long ago, I naively thought that we could actually measure neural activity directly, but what we're actually measuring is just the blood flow—the change in the amount of blood supplying energy to those regions that need it because they're the ones that are currently active.

UF: That's right. But as you say it's several steps down the road to get to the activity in the neurons. We are really at the beginning of this exciting new discovery of the mind, of the brain, how the brain works. We just don't know it yet.

It's very comparable, I think, to astronomers in the early 17th century when they first developed telescopes to look at the night sky and could suddenly see many things for the first time.

But they still couldn't see very well, and it was simply a time where you could only guess what might be out there. And it would have been absurd to say: *"Well, all that's there is what we can see through these lenses at the moment."*

I think the same will happen in the discovery of the mind. We now know it's possible to get there, we now know that there are many ways we can increase our understanding.

There are those, of course, who start from the other side, the molecular end: they look at a single cell, a single neuron, taken from, say, a rat brain or something like that. They learn what goes in and what goes out, how cells signal to each other, and how those, in turn, develop into large-scale brain networks.

It's very impressive that we know in principle how cells work, how synapses work. But at the other level of cognitive neuroscience we are still trying to find out how our thoughts are represented in the brain.

HB: I guess the goal is to have these two levels meet.

UF: I think that's the exciting thing. It's like digging a huge tunnel, where you should really bear in mind that you are doing it from both ends. It seems to me at the moment that there is sometimes a lack of awareness that we are all working together in this whole enterprise.

I think there is sometimes too much enthusiasm to stress one perspective at the expense of the other. Some will say, *"We'll get there from bottom up!"* You know: single cell, then two cells together, gradually building things up and getting more complicated.

Meanwhile the other side is saying, *"Forget about all that: if we talk about feelings, if we talk about mentalizing, these are big concepts and you can't map them to single cells in neurons: it's millions, billions."*

They are all somehow connected to each other in very strange ways that we don't quite understand. So the two sides are not yet joining up but I think they will.

HB: I imagine that when you started your research career in psychology the idea that we would ever be able to have a real-time look at any living brain must have seemed almost like science fiction.

UF: That's absolutely right. We did, of course, rely very much on neuropsychological data from naturally occurring lesions in the brain. That gave some kind of insight into how specialized certain parts of the brain are for things like language or vision, which enabled us to further distance ourselves from the idea of this dualism of mind and brain.

After all, if some bit of the brain has been lesioned by some accident, by some trauma, it's clearly not mind over matter any more. You just have to accept this.

Brain-imaging technology has had an enormous impact. One of the frustrating things in these developmental neurological conditions, where something is slightly different from birth, is that there is nothing obviously drastically different: there is no lesion. Even now when people look at the brain post-mortem in autism, it's very difficult to pinpoint exactly what's critically different.

After all, every single brain is different. And now we have this huge spectrum of autism, so there are an enormous number of differences due to all sorts of things; not only intelligence but also potential differences between males and females, potential differences in ages and what sort of compensatory learning is involved, personality, temperament and so on.

But eventually, as the technology improves, you should be able to see all of these differences in some kind of physiological sense in the brain. We're not there yet, but we will get there.

Questions for Discussion:

1. How do you think brain-imaging technology will change in the next 10, 20 and 50 years?

2. Are there moral and ethical risks associated with a drastic improvement in brain-scanning technology? If so, what, exactly, should be done to reduce them?

V. Vaccines

Correlation vs. causation

HB: I'd like to talk about something a little bit different now. We've talked extensively of your ideas of "theory of mind" and "mentalizing", the behavioural experiments that support your views, as well as the brain-imaging studies that provide neurobiological evidence in terms of specific brain networks associated with these concepts.

Earlier, you mentioned that you believe autism to be a developmental disorder. Reading through the literature, it seems that the symptoms characteristic of autism typically do not normally appear until the child's second year, around 18 months or something like that.

So there is an understandable sense of panic and desolation that a parent will have when first confronted with the prospect of an autistic child. Everything seemed to be going along swimmingly and then all of a sudden something seems to happen when the child is roughly around 18 months or so. Is that a fair description of what often happens?

UF: Yes, I think so.

HB: Hence the believe in autism being a developmental disorder. We can talk about the genetic underpinnings of all of this, but at this point I'm putting myself in the perspective of a fraught parent, who would have a natural tendency to say something like, "*My child was completely healthy up until this point,*" and suddenly all these odd behavioural traits start surfacing. Under the circumstances, there would be a natural tendency to start looking for environmental factors that might have triggered things.

UF: There is, yes.

HB: And as you and others have written about, some people were of the view that vaccinations were to blame. In particular there is a triple vaccination for measles, mumps and rubella that was singled out.

UF: That's right. That was one that was blamed for an increase in autism.

HB: Right. So you can certainly understand the chain of reasoning that led to that: *"My child looked to be fine. And this specific thing happened at the time when they first started to show symptoms: they were vaccinated with this particular triple vaccine."*
   This naturally led to a great fear that this vaccination was somehow responsible for autism. And my understanding is that people did careful studies about this.

UF: Yes: they did careful studies. It had to be taken seriously as a hypothesis. It needed to be investigated and it was. And it was absolutely not supported by study after study, but it took an incredibly long time to convince people that this was just not true.
   It was just one of these many hypotheses that are worth considering and investigating. It turned out to be a blind alley and you've got to reject it. But there are still people who won't accept that even now: they're just so completely wedded to this idea that that's what must have happened.

HB: Yet there is no shred of scientific evidence for it whatsoever.

UF: There is no scientific evidence for it at all. It's not because there was some kind of denial, some kind of effort to hide problems having to do with the use of vaccinations which is so very beneficial for all of us—

HB: So there's no conspiracy.

UF: There is no conspiracy.

HB: In short: there is no scientific evidence for it; it's just wrong. It's a plausible hypothesis that turned out to be wrong.

UF: Yes: a hypothesis that just turned out to be wrong, exactly. Of course, we have to acknowledge that as human beings we want to have explanations: we need to know why something happened.

HB: Particularly if it's one's child.

UF: Absolutely. And this is still going on. There are still ideas that are often very outlandish and you suddenly say: "*My God, can people really think that **this** could cause autism in their child?*" Well, there is such a great desire to have something to hang on to, possibly something that exonerates you in some sense from blame.

We have to turn to a biological basis, to a genetic basis, in the end. There's an enormous amount of research going on that shows that there isn't just *one* gene responsible for autism, there isn't even a handful of genes that's responsible, there isn't even knowledge about particular genes that would account for *all* of autism: it seems that each bit of autism of this whole spectrum has its own causes.

Some look at the situation through the perspective of genetic mutations: there's a mutation that happens in the sperm, for example, or in the egg, and that's what leads to autism. That can happen. But again, it's only a minority of cases where any such pathway has been explicitly demonstrated. It won't be true for all cases.

HB: But however complicated and abstruse the particular genetic mechanism or mechanisms may be—maybe we won't understand them for 100 years or more—we *do* have considerable confidence that there *is* a genetic mechanism underlying this condition, as opposed to something environmental, be it a vaccine or something else.

UF: Exactly.

HB: So we don't really have to pay too much attention worrying about any other possible environmental trigger?

UF: Yes, that's what I believe. There are toxins and other factors that might play some role in combination with a given genetic predisposition but not independent of the predisposition itself.

Predisposition is what it's all about: probabilities. All the genetic research shows that even if you have the predisposition you don't necessarily have to get whatever that predisposes you for because there might be mitigating factors, there might be ways of making you particularly resilient.

So you don't necessarily have to have a sort of fatalistic view which says, "*Nothing can be done about it.*" That doesn't follow from thinking about these genetic causes.

There are ways of thinking about this as a very complex interplay of rather random factors that might happen; that might make things better for some, worse for others. All sorts of hazards can happen during early neural development; it's a very complex story.

It's quite obvious that most cognitive faculties can be totally intact and functioning well in people who nonetheless can't easily mentalize and show other additional signs of autism.

So it's something incredibly subtle. It's not like having a non-viable organism, it's not like that: it's a good brain. And many people are arguing that it's very wrong to see it as an abnormality or disease or disorder because it is such a subtle thing that it really falls under normal personality variations.

HB: Presumably that has something to do with, again, the level of autism that we are talking about.

UF: I think so, yes.

HB: Since there is such a wide variety of people who suffer from autism, or who are involved in autism spectrum disorder, you have people who are, as we had mentioned, formally classified as mentally retarded who presumably have serious impairments in functioning in their day-to-day life. Then on the other end of the spectrum you have clearly very intelligent people, some of whom have been diagnosed with Asperger syndrome.

UF: Yes, right.

HB: As you mentioned in one of your books, Hans Asperger himself was of the view that there was some clear correlation between this condition and those who were capable of works of genius in the arts and sciences. Is that a fair summary?

UF: Yes, I think that's an absolutely correct summary. And from that part of the spectrum you really cannot but think: *Yes, we are talking about some kind of personality variation.*

There is a huge heterogeneity in the individual lives of human beings, and you cannot say one is better than the other or one is healthier than the other: that's absolute nonsense. And what we at the moment call 'autistic' or 'autistic-like' is perhaps part of this personality variation.

But I think there is a difference for those cases where there is possibly much suffering, not only for the individuals but for their families as well. I think to dismiss that lightly by just saying, "*Oh, that's just a personality variation*", is not right. It's actually important to really concentrate and say how can we help these families.

It's very interesting that so much learning can happen. It's very encouraging to recognize that even if you have a child who has a lot of severe problems that sometimes go together with autism—like having very little language, being very uncoordinated, having attention deficits and generally being very limited in daily activities—even then, you can do a lot about that with appropriate programs. There are good techniques available, good practices.

But, again, here is an area where the quacks come in, the charlatans who single out their own programs for praise. So parents have to be very aware that they should *only* go for those programs where there is some scientific basis, where there is some evidence that they can say, "*Yes, that has been shown to be good*" and not be taken in by people who promise unhelpful things. And that does include the psychoanalysis.

HB: I'd like to come back to the question of specific advice to parents and families at the end, but there are a few more issues I'd like to discuss first.

UF: Of course. So far we've only considered the social aspects at the core of autism. We haven't really considered the non-social aspects.

Questions for Discussion:

1. Why do you think that a substantial number of people are adamant that there is a global conspiracy to "cover up" a link between autism and childhood vaccines? Is there anything that might convince them otherwise?

2. Is there a danger of looking at every medical condition as merely some sort of "human variation"? Where should we draw the line?

3. What role should government play in protecting the public from the "quacks and charlatans" that Uta warns us against?

VI. Probing the Spectrum

Big and little pictures

HB: Before I get to the non-social aspects of autism, I want to briefly talk about something else in the public consciousness, something we've already mentioned in passing, which is this expression "Asperger syndrome".

UF: Oh, yes.

HB: I don't know what it is.

UF: OK.

HB: Earlier we were talking about the spectrum associated with autism, and I appreciate that those diagnosed with Asperger's are typically on the extremely intelligent side of the spectrum, and I know that Hans Asperger was one of the founders of autism, but none of that makes it terribly clear to me what Asperger syndrome actually *is*.

I'd also like to spend a bit of time talking about something that is also generally associated with autism: this notion of the savant, the *Rain Man* type of character who, while being terribly dysfunctional in many ways, has these incredible areas of expertise and ability.

But first, perhaps you can give me a definition of what Asperger syndrome is.

UF: Asperger syndrome is something that has a slightly slippery definition that changes, and at the moment it's coming out of favour, unfortunately.

HB: It is? I didn't realize that. Why is that?

UF: Well, Asperger syndrome, quite briefly, is really a form of autism. So the question is: "*Why shouldn't you just call it autism?*" And at the moment there's a big trend to say, "*Let's call it autism.*"

HB: Just for the sake of completeness.

UF: Yes. Given that the autistic spectrum is so very wide, it's perfectly fine to say, "*This is also autism*" and not give it that separate label. But the label *does* do an interesting job and serves an interesting purpose: it tells you that it's perfectly possible not to have any learning disability, possess really fluent language and still have the features of autism.

The features of autism being: problems communicating, difficulties with mentalizing, having a concentration on narrow, stereotypical interests, exhibiting a kind of repetitive behaviour and being somewhat set and rigid in your life.

All of this sometimes comes together as a package, personified by a child who is a "little professor": perhaps someone who has amazing ability in playing chess and beats even the very experienced adults; talks in a language that's extraordinarily advanced for his age but doesn't play with other children, and isn't interested in joining up with typical child-like games. Maybe he is also very narrow in his interests: only passionate about chess and not anything else and being—well, not quite like other children, but even in a good sense— where parents might feel rightly proud of their"little genius".

This idea of having a little genius when you have an autistic child, that's the idea that's been used in practically all the movies that have been made about autism. It started with *Rain Man* in 1988 that portrayed autism in a very truthful way in one sense, but also in a totally romantic and exaggerated way in other ways.

As you know, the *Rain Man* character had these incredible savant skills. That is, of course, something pretty rare to the extent that he possessed them. Savant skills by themselves are not that rare, but what is generally meant by that is having elevated abilities that are superior to others: memory ability, reading ability, musical ability, and so on. But the sort of "world beating" memory excellence displayed by the *Rain Man* character is very rare and you can't assume that that's typical of any autistic person or any Asperger person that you will meet.

They *do* exist, these exceptionally prodigious savants who are kind of *wonders of the world*; and they are extremely interesting. And it seems to me that they all have autism. It's not that you can be like that and not have all these other features of being sort of single-minded and not so interested in your peers and social communication.

But these people also show how much they like to be in this social sphere, how they thrive on the attention they get—they actually show you that they are really fun people,; they are very nice and very engaging.

You can watch videos of them and see how they thrive on being fêted, on being nurtured in this particular way.

This also happens with the other cases who are not such outstanding fantastic talents. And you *do* find some kind of talent in many cases, I believe. I think that was one of the great puzzles that needed to be explained: how the mind can work in such a way that some things seem to be so good—these feats of memory, for example—and yet at the same time this memory wasn't used in order to get meaning from the world.

This led to one of the theories that I pursued, one which has also, I think, stood the test of time, although it is less accepted than the mentalizing theory. I call it "weak central coherence", on the grounds that we have a natural striving to normally make sense of the world in this sort of big way, in a very holistic way, going to meaning in ever bigger ways. That seems to be a kind of drive we put in our information processing system.

HB: To look at the bigger picture.

UF: To look at the bigger picture, not minding if you have to lose the detail. That I would call "strong central coherence": everything should cohere, something should be there.

But there is, again, a considerable amount of individual variation, and there are people who are not going for this. They are going for the detail, they are going for the actual, truthful, verbatim factual things and for them the overall meaning is not such an overriding concern.

At least those were my thoughts at the very beginning of the development of the theory. It has since shifted in quite interesting ways so that now I believe that there's a balance: perhaps you can switch from being holistic to detailed, or from detailed to holistic.

At this point in time I think it may be a theory that can be applied only to a subgroup of this autism spectrum, but it's an interesting subgroup because the ones who are really interested in details seem very likely to have some kind of savant skill that has to do with that detail, such as finding embedded figures where other people can't see them, or this particularly excellent memory for verbatim detail: noticing changes in the environment which you and I would probably overlook completely.

This is the kind of mind that's somehow able to set aside the sort of illusions or distractions that might otherwise appear to us through our more holistic perception.

HB: You give a wonderful example: a type of puzzle where some types of autistic children can do the puzzle independent of the overall picture.

UF: That's exactly right. I found that absolutely astonishing but true: they can really do it without looking at the overall picture.

HB: So you could even turn it over, have it all blank and they're just looking at the shapes: they're not being guided by the overall picture at all. They're processing information quite differently.

UF: Yes. This is a different style of information processing and many have actually argued, particularly my collaborators—in particular Francesca Happé—that it's a style of information processing which is totally distributed in the normal population.

So you can find that sort of thing in people who are not autistic, they're just like that: they can do these jigsaw puzzles upside down and there is nothing autistic about them. Her argument is, "*Yes, it does coincide with a sort of classic autism but it's a separate personality dimension which has nothing to do, in a sort of neurological genetic origin, with the mentalizing problem."*

HB: But it seems to me that those are two different statements. One statement is that there is a broad spectrum of basic human orientation: there is the super-detailed orientation on one side and the super-Gestalt, big-picture orientation on the other side, and all human beings fall somewhere in this spectrum.

UF: Most fall in the middle. And most can do both.

HB: Right. But my point is that such a statement seems quite a different thing than saying, *"Be that as it may, the overwhelming statistical majority of autism individuals happen to fall over here in this particularly narrow range."*

UF: Yes.

HB: That seems like that's suggestive of something.

UF: But it could be just historical: that these things stood out together and we'll actually find that we can separate them out and may eventually determine different, more meaningful, diagnostic categories.

At the moment, I believe the diagnostic categories are too unwieldy, too wide. They're not useful as they are, and we will have to come to these sub-categories but we don't know what they should be yet. But this could be a kind of guidance.

I mean, I know exactly what the classic autistic child should be like as originally described by the psychologist Leo Kanner: the child who has this aloofness, isn't connecting to this world, and who also has some stereotyped behaviours—he's very rigid and also some kind of relatively outstanding ability.

Now that package I recognize. The question is: *"Is that package due to the same kind of underlying processes that produce this? Or is it a sort of coincidence?"*

I say a "sort of coincidence" because I've actually rejected the idea that it's a *complete* coincidence. But at any rate, we just don't know yet: we don't know yet whether this is a particular subgroup about which we should say, "*OK, that's the Kanner type.*"

The Asperger type is actually very similar except it seems all much milder, much more to do with good language while the Kanner type has to do with bad language—on the whole, very, very impaired language.

Again, people say: "*Why don't you explain that specifically, this impaired language?*" And you could say: "*OK, that's another add-on: it's a superimposed thing that you happen to get.*"

You're on this hazardous developmental path: one thing has gone wrong already, another thing has gone wrong. Now we come to language: that could be going wrong in many different ways too...

We've tried to explain the language difficulties in terms of lack of mentalizing but that doesn't fit with the Asperger-type where language problems *don't* occur but the mentalizing problems do. There could be degrees of this mentalizing ability, we don't yet know. At the moment, that's quite difficult to think about—we haven't got, I suppose, quite refined enough behavioural tests. People are thinking quite hard about what we could do to really clarify the kind of degrees you might have.

People have said: "*Isn't it the case that ordinary individuals differ in their theory of mind, in this mentalizing?*" Well, in terms of how consciously they can successfully be Machiavellian or not, absolutely. That must be so. But in terms of this intuitive innate thing, I think that's just the same for everybody.

HB: It seems to me there is an equal danger in the other direction, that is, not acknowledging clear statistical correlations and instead simply saying, "*Well, everybody's different.*"

UF: Yes, it's very tricky. There are these discussions that have been going on ever since I can remember: "*How can you say that somebody is mad? I mean, aren't we all? Aren't we all a little bit mad? Think how demeaning it must be to put that label on to somebody!*"

HB: Especially when it comes to people who are highly active and highly creative.

UF: Exactly. Once again, I think it's all still a legacy of dualism, which says: "*Here is the body and the brain, and there is the mind, which is completely separate. The mind can't really be ill like the body can be ill, or have something missing like the body can have something missing.*"

I'm not talking about something vital to our survival, but something you can manage without: you can live with one kidney, you can live with less than ten fingers.

I think the same applies to the mind. And whether you call something "normal" or "abnormal"—well, you have to get used to it. I mean, we can say, "*It's not normal not to have ten fingers.*" But we don't have to necessarily look down upon people who, through no choice of their own, are born with less than ten fingers.

Questions for Discussion:

1. Can certain activities (such as politics or history) be regarded as being more naturally "Gestalt-oriented", while others are more "detail oriented" (like mathematics or chess)?

2. Do you agree or disagree with the idea that a child diagnosed with Asperger syndrome should simply be regarded as "autistic"? Why or why not?

VII. Gender

A provocative speculation

HB: Another thing that I was surprised to learn about autism was that there is a huge asymmetry in the number of diagnosed cases between boys and girls.

UF: Yes.

HB: So one can attribute all sorts of possible explanations for this, but it seems to me that if the sample size is large enough and if this has been happening for a long enough period of time, that's indicative of *something* neurologically in terms of the distinction between men and women.

UF: Absolutely.

HB: And to deny that on the basis of: *"Oh no, we must all be exactly the same, because that's my philosophical belief "* or something—

UF: That's not scientific.

HB: Right. And here's something I'm going to say which might be a little bit provocative and outlandish, because we've been chatting for a while and it seems time for me to go out on a limb.

UF: OK, good. Go ahead.

HB: Well, I used to run a theoretical physics institute. And theoretical physics, as most people know, is a discipline that happens to be highly male-dominated.

So I'm not a psychologist, nor do I pretend to be one, but it seems pretty clear to me that if you look at the characteristic profiles of individuals who are in this field—on average, statistically—you find a pretty strong overlap between many of the characteristics that you've been describing with respect to Asperger syndrome.

These tend to be people who are highly intelligent and highly analytical, but oriented towards very specific tasks that can sometimes be of a pretty repetitive nature. They are clearly gifted at what they're doing, but as a rule they're not terribly interested in anything outside of their small area of specialization.

So when I read about the preponderance of male cases of autism over female cases, I thought, *Isn't that interesting—there seems to be a correlation here that is suggestive of...well, **something**.

Obviously this is all anecdotal and I haven't done any rigorous studies, but it would seem to me to be criminally unscientific to simply ignore what strikes me as a fairly obvious correlation that I've witnessed so many times with my own eyes and just refuse to consider investigating it more rigorously.

UF: Absolutely. I completely agree and there are, of course, labs all over the world that are really starting from that point and trying to make some sense of things; that's being actively researched.

There could be different reasons like in the chromosomes or in hormones or in the level of testosterone prenatally. Anything like that could give some causes that lead to these kinds of differences and that give you these interesting overlaps between types of personalities that choose to be theoretical physicists or mathematicians.

And yes, I do agree that this is very provocative and very interesting. I would say that these physicists and mathematicians being detail-focused and very rigid and not interested in many aspects of social interaction probably could all do the intuitive mentalizing tasks if they were given them. That is a bet. I would think the experiment should be done.

HB: Well, it's an open question, I tell you.

UF: OK, it's an open question. But it's not all there is to autism. It is certainly one particular thing, which is actually such a bad thing that I don't think you could be a very successful experimental physicist unless—

HB: Oh, not the experimentalists. The experimentalists are fine.

UF: OK, so then theoretical physicists. But I think it would make it really difficult to succeed if they were really in that category.

HB: Perhaps.

Questions for Discussion:

1. Were you aware of the fact that many more boys than girls are diagnosed as autistic? Why do you think that might be?

2. Might the very notion of "success" in certain detail-oriented disciplines like theoretical physics be dependent on the psychological orientation of its practitioners?

VIII. Ways Forward

Some concrete approaches

HB: I'd like to now return to something that I promised to talk more about earlier. I'd like to return to the perspective of the anxious parent who has an autistic child.

We've been talking about ways in which one can define autism, we've talked about neurological studies, we've talked about experimental psychological studies, we've talked about theories that might explain it, we've tried to pin things down sufficiently while naturally hesitating about being too sweeping in our generalizations.

UF: Right.

HB: But let's say my son Johnny here has recently been diagnosed as autistic, and I'm obviously very worried. I'm now convinced that the root cause is not environmental, and I understand that this is a genetic disorder, a neurological developmental disorder.

But what am I going to do now? You've got all this knowledge from all these years of studying this: how can you help make his life and my life better? I know what I shouldn't do: I know I shouldn't feel guilty or trek off to a Freudian to hear what a terrible non-bonding mother I've been…

UF: That's already a very good step.

More generally, I think the theories that psychologists like me have devised do allow for some way into the situation to gain a certain measure of understanding.

If you can use such knowledge and say: "*OK, this is what I can expect, this is what I can't expect*", you are already moving in a more positive direction.

And there are many schemes available: teaching autistic children social situations where they can become familiar with what other people might think, what perspectives they might have that are different, why they might have certain feelings, and how the feelings are expressed. These programs seem to be really working.

HB: So they're learning by example?

UF: They're learning by patient repetition, in a typical way that you would teach a child who is not naturally able to do maths, for example, who really seems to have some kind of neurological problems doing numbers. You can still teach that child very patiently, in different ways, something like algebra, geometry, all sorts of things.

HB: You can teach by analogy too, I imagine.

UF: Yes. You might have to accept certain limitations—it depends on the strengths and weaknesses of the child.

So again, by analogy with a child who hasn't got a number sense, who can't ever really get his head around bigger numbers, smaller numbers, subtraction and so forth, he can still learn a lot by heart, by rote to just get there anyway. And he can use a calculator, just like we can use apps for all sorts of things nowadays.

In fact, there are lots of apps available now that have been especially created for the autistic community, by parents or by autistic people themselves.

They can rely on the ability to concentrate and focus on something, to repeat, if necessary, a task that's quite difficult, as long as it's enjoyably done with some kind of reward at the end. But very often being able to play a computer game is a reward in itself. Indeed, you find many cases that the autistic child is not actually socially averse or aloof, but that they have social interests and social interaction in this very basic sense that we all have: they like to be the centre of attention.

HB: But they may not know how to do it.

UF: They need to have the techniques on how to not put off other people.

For example, it's often important to explain to an autistic child that he should look at other people—not necessarily in the eyes, that's another matter; they might really, genuinely, not like to do that—but to vaguely look in their direction and to smile. You can teach all of these things, which might make it much easier for the other person who may not know anything about autism to get a kind of conversation going.

They are often so eager to learn to understand other people, they really will work very, very hard. These programs are available, these techniques are available. There are also techniques that are based on learning psychology that have quite a good scientific basis on how to control difficult behaviour, how to make certain things easier, even how to improve language and speech. Many different problems have their own solutions; and of course some are more important than others.

But on the whole, I feel really very optimistic just looking at the kinds of programs that are available. And the best thing of all, actually, is that there is a very active community that networks exceptionally well. That has been extremely good and beneficial, and I hope that it will continue.

Of course, there's always a danger of the charlatans preying on that community. So as long as one is extra suspicious and extra careful about that, I think it's really good to have that mutual help and understanding.

The point is not to declare: "*I'm not going to rest until my child is completely indistinguishable from any other child.*" That would not be a reasonable aim of the exercise, but rather instead do your utmost to nurture the strengths that are there while taking into account the weaknesses, just like you would with any other child.

HB: As you said earlier, this is a developmental disorder. Presumably there are limits, depending on the child and depending on the circumstances—as there are for all of us—but just because one has a developmental disorder hardly means that one can't continue to learn and improve.

UF: Absolutely. A great example of this is someone like Temple Grandin, who is autistic and such a dynamic and impressive personality. She says that she learns all the time. She's now over 60 and still learning, still impressing you with new skills that she's developed.

HB: Well, I've certainly learned an enormous amount from this discussion and had a wonderful time as well. Thanks so much for chatting with me, Uta.

UF: My pleasure. Thank you for your interest.

Question for Discussion:

1. How has this conversation changed your perspective of autism? What would you have liked to have seen discussed more? Less?

Continuing the Conversation

Readers are encouraged to read Uta's books, *Autism: Explaining the Enigma* and *Autism: A Very Short Introduction*, which naturally go into considerable additional detail about many of the issues discussed here.

Ideas Roadshow has two other conversations that deal explicitly with the subject of autism: *Our Human Variability* with Stephen Scherer and *Autism: A Genetic Perspective* with Jay Gargus.

Ideas Roadshow Collections

Each Ideas Roadshow collection offers 5 separate expert conversations presented in an accessible and engaging format.

- *Conversations About Anthropology & Sociology*
- *Conversations About Astrophysics & Cosmology*
- *Conversations About Biology*
- *Conversations About History, Volume 1*
- *Conversations About History, Volume 2*
- *Conversations About History, Volume 3*
- *Conversations About Language & Culture*
- *Conversations About Law*
- *Conversations About Neuroscience*
- *Conversations About Philosophy, Volume 1*
- *Conversations About Philosophy, Volume 2*
- *Conversations About Physics, Volume 1*
- *Conversations About Physics, Volume 2*
- *Conversations About Politics*
- *Conversations About Psychology, Volume 1*
- *Conversations About Psychology, Volume 2*
- *Conversations About Religion*
- *Conversations About Social Psychology*
- *Conversations About The Environment*
- *Conversations About The History of Ideas*

All collections are available as both eBook and paperback.

* 9 7 8 1 7 7 1 7 0 1 7 1 6 *